D1557649

Springer Series: THE TEACHING OF NURSING

Series Editor: Diane O. McGivern, RN, PhD, FAAN

Advisory Board: *Ellen Baer, PhD, RN, FAAN; Carla Mariano, EdD, RN; Janet A. Rodgers, PhD, RN, FAAN; Alice Adam Young, PhD, RN*

Patricia A. Bailey, Ed.D., R.N., C.S., is Professor of Nursing and Director of the Service-Learning Program in the Department of Nursing at the University of Scranton, Scranton, Pennsylvania. Her research focus has been on academic integrity of students, professional identity, and service-learning. She is the recipient of several awards and grants. In 1997 she received the Distinguished Service Award from the College of Health, Education and Human Resources at the University of Scranton. In 1998 she was one of 10 national finalists for the Campus Compact 1998 Ehrlich Award for Service-Learning.

Dona Rinaldi Carpenter, Ed.D., R.N., C.S., is Professor of Nursing and Director of the RN-BS Track at the University of Scranton, Scranton, Pennsylvania. She teaches medical-surgical nursing and research in the undergraduate and graduate curriculum. Her research interests focus on qualitative methods, doctoral education in nursing, professional commitment, and quality of life. She has authored and co-authored several books, articles, and book chapters and has presented her research at national and international conferences. Dr. Carpenter has co-authored a text on qualitative research with Dr. Helen J. Streubert, which received the American Journal of Nursing Book of the Year Award in 1995.

Patricia A. Harrington, Ed.D., R.N., C.S., is Assistant Professor and Chairperson of the Department of Nursing at the University of Scranton, Scranton, Pennsylvania. In addition to chairing the department, she teaches Pathophysiology, Nursing Fundamentals and Maternity Nursing. Her research investigations have included mother-infant relationships in teenagers and HIV prevention and outreach. She is the recipient of several service awards from the American Red Cross for her work in HIV prevention education.

Integrating Community Service into Nursing Education

A Guide to Service-Learning

Patricia A. Bailey, EdD, RN, CS
Dona Rinaldi Carpenter, EdD, RN, CS
Patricia A. Harrington, EdD, RN, CS
Editors

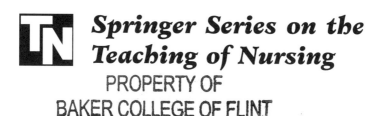

Springer Series on the Teaching of Nursing

Copyright © 1999 by Springer Publishing Company, Inc.

Springer Publishing Company, Inc.
536 Broadway
New York, NY 10012–3955

Acquisition Editor: Ruth Chasek
Production Editor: Sandi Borger
Cover design by Janet Joachim

99 00 01 02   03 / 5 4 3 2 1

Library of Congress Cataloging-in-Publication Data

Integrating community service into nursing education : a guide to service-
  learning / Patricia A. Bailey, Dona Rinaldi Carpenter, and Patricia A.
  Harrington, editors.
      p.   cm. — (Springer series, the teaching of nursing)
    Includes bibliographical references and index.
    ISBN 0-8261-1268-4 (hardcover)
    1. Nursing—In—service training. 2. Nursing—Study and teaching
  (Continuing education) 3. Social service. I. Bailey, Patricia A. (Patricia
  Ann). II. Carpenter, Dona Rinaldi. III. Harrington, Patricia A.
  IV. Series: Springer series on the teaching of nursing.
    [DNLM: 1. Education, Nursing. 2. Altruism. 3. Community-
  Institutional Relations. 4. Curriculum. 5. Voluntary Workers.
  WY 18 1597 1999]
  RT76.I55   1999
  610.73'071'55—dc21
  DNLM/DLC
  for Library of Congress   99-26341
                                                                 CIP

Printed in the United States of America

This book is dedicated to our students and to our community partners. Students are at the heart of what we do as educators. Our opportunities to expand and have impact on their learning while preparing them for life-long leadership only exist because of their open, curious natures. Their commitment to developing a strong service-learning program is evidenced by their willingness to go above and beyond the call of duty in terms of working, evaluating, and refining the service-learning component of our curriculum. They have taught us the importance of remaining curious, committed, and concerned about all aspects of our world.

To our community partners we say thank you from the bottom of our hearts. Without your willingness to take a risk, try something different, and commit to new and emerging ideas, service-learning would not exist. We appreciate the fact that you trusted us and took us into your world, allowing our students and faculty to grow and learn in ways that would not have been otherwise possible.

Contents

List of Contributors

Peggy Begley, Volunteer Director
Visiting Nurse Association, Hospice of Lackawanna County
301 Delaware Street
Olyphant, PA 18447

Janet Moskovitz, Volunteer Coordinator
The Jewish Home of Eastern Pennsylvania
1101 Vine Street
Scranton, PA 18510

Candal B. Sakevich, Women's Outreach Coordinator
Wyoming Valley Chapter American Red Cross
Women's Outreach Program
156 South Franklin Street
Wilkes-Barre, PA 18701

Tracy Lyn Svalina, Director, Health Services
Scranton Chapter American Red Cross
545 Jefferson Avenue
Scranton, PA 18510

Preface

Service-learning has many definitions based on how the service program is structured in a particular institution. However in general, service-learning can be defined as a structured learning experience which combines community service with student preparation and reflection. A connecting link is established between academics and service. A definition of service-learning that was published by the National and Community Service Trust Act of 1993 focuses on essential components of service-learning which include: learning and developing through organized service activities that are meeting identified community needs. Service activities should foster civic responsibility, be incorporated into the academic curriculum and provide opportunity to reflect on experiences individually and in groups. The service-learning program described in this text is based on these essential components, namely, that students learn and develop, needs of the community are met, relationships exist between the community and the University, civic responsibility is encouraged, service is centered in the curriculum, and reflection takes place.

Consider the following situations: a group of students presents an HIV/AIDS education program to area high school students; a student spends time as a volunteer with a local inpatient hospice program; several students who are involved in sports programs on campus spend their Saturday mornings teaching basketball skills to children at a local Boy's and Girls' Club. What are these students doing? They are engaged in a service-learning program that is a course requirement and are being asked to reflect on their experiences in light of course objectives and personal experiences. They are learning in the community setting, meeting community needs and achieving course objectives.

The central focus of this textbook is the integration of service-learning into the nursing curriculum. The components of service-learning and its central relationship to education and curriculum are addressed. Issues related to service-learning with narrative comments from some of the 300 students who have participated in service-learning to date have been incorporated.

Clearly, our resources for life and health are more and more community centered. Instilling a sense of community in those individuals being prepared at the college level can facilitate a sense of responsibility and ensure their commitment to give back to their community over the course of their careers in healthcare.

This book is intended to be a beginning dialogue for the development and initiation of service-learning programs in the nursing curriculum. The text is organized to facilitate the reader's comprehension of the fundamental approaches to incorporating service-learning. Not only does this book focus on the nuts and bolts of initiating a service-learning program but it is also rich with descriptions of the life experiences of college students who have participated in service-learning. In Chapter 1, "The Concept of Service-Learning," the reader is introduced to the basic components of a service-learning program and its defining characteristics. The historical roots of service-learning are explored and related to the current state of service-learning throughout the nation. The various definitions that have been developed and their relationships to a true service-learning program are reviewed.

In Chapter 2, "Integrating Service-Learning into the Curriculum," important ingredients for a successful service-learning program are described. Lessons learned during the first three years of a new service-learning program are described along with strategies for trouble-shooting. Concrete examples and suggestions for incorporating service-learning into the nursing curriculum are provided.

Chapter 3, "Critical Reflection," explores various technologies for guiding students in the reflection process, an essential component of the service-learning experience. Activities such as journaling, reaction papers, and classroom reflection are discussed in detail with examples of student reflections about their service-learning experience.

Chapter 4 addresses the "Promises and Problems" that are encountered when implementing a service-learning program. The rewards of service-learning are reviewed, while potential pitfalls are discussed in reference to each aspect of a service-learning program.

In Chapter 5, "Community Partnerships in Service-Learning" focuses on the importance of establishing strong ties with the community in the form of partnerships which will enhance student learning and facilitate the goal of meeting the needs of the local community. Examples of the impact service-learning had on four community agencies participating in the service-learning program described in this text are also included.

The appendices conclude the text and offer helpful information regarding service-learning resources, quantitative and qualitative evaluation forms and samples of actual course integration of a service-learning program. This text should serve as a resource for the integration of service-learning into the nursing curriculum. Creativity and perseverance are the keys to beginning. Commitment and on-going evaluation will see new programs brought to fruition.

The examples of service-learning included in this book are drawn from the program that provides the basic framework presented. This program was developed in 1995, when the program was funded by a three-year grant from the Health Professions Schools in Service to the Nation, a program of the Pew Health Professions Commission and the National Fund for Medical Education, with support from the Pew Charitable Trusts, the Corporation for National Service, and the Health Resources and Services Administration.

One of the most "helpful" lessons learned from a service-learning program is that there are many ways to integrate a service component into the curriculum. The individual needs of the program and the community structure in which the program operates will influence the direction service-learning takes. It is essential that there is institutional support for a program before one attempts to approach faculty. Strong institutional support and faculty development will pave the way for a successful service-learning program. Clear direction to students and on-going education regarding the goals and purposes of service-learning will assist students to value the benefits of service, remain involved and motivated, and to see the connections to learning.

Acknowledgments

The authors wish to acknowledge the commitment of nursing students, faculty and administration, all of whom have contributed to the success of the service-learning initiative that began at the University of Scranton Department of Nursing in 1995. Without the support of all nursing faculty, the opportunity to incorporate service-learning into required nursing courses would have remained a dream. The nursing faculty answered the challenge and facilitated student interest in service-learning and supported the program through their own role-modeling of community service.

Specifically, we wish to acknowledge those who have been most closely involved in the initiation of the program and the production of this text. First and foremost, we would like to acknowledge Serena D. Seifer, M.D., Program Director, and Kara Connors, Program Coordinator, of the Health Professions Schools in Service to the Nation Program (HPSISN) whose guidance and direction were essential and contributed to the success of our service-learning program; Barbara Holland, Ph.D., co-director of the HPSISN evaluation team, for thoughtful critique and continued support of our service-learning program; Patricia Vaccaro, B.A., M.S., Director of Collegiate Volunteers at the University of Scranton, whose support, enthusiasm, and willingness to go above and beyond the call of duty facilitated the successful incorporation of service-learning in the nursing curriculum; Andrea Malone, research assistant and graduate of the class of 1998, for her precision and attention to detail while helping with the literature review for this text; a special thank-you to Cara Catalino, Ann Marie Ryan, and Sally Ann Quiterio, nursing majors at the University of Scranton, for their work on the advisory committee and participation in national conferences as student representatives; Virginia Morrison, R.N., M.S., and Cathy Champi, R.N., B.S., graduate assistants working directly with the service-learning program, whose community connections and excellent people skills facilitated the program's development; Dr. James Pallante, Dean of the J.A. Panuska College of Professional Studies, who was responsible for inspiring the idea of student service and who has supported all our efforts to integrate service-learning into the nursing curriculum; and Dr. Richard Passon, Academic Vice-President/Provost, for his unwavering support and interest in the development of service-learning. Lastly, we wish to thank our former President of the University, Rev. J.A. Panuska, S.J., who has helped faculty, staff, and students see the importance of "service" in all its dimensions. His commitment to the Mission of the University, namely, to "prepare men and women to serve others," has structured a foundation for our service-learning program. His encouragement and support has been greatly appreciated, and his wisdom and gentle guidance will never be forgotten.

CHAPTER 1

The Concept of Service-Learning

Dona Rinaldi Carpenter, Ed.D., R.N., C.S.

> I believe learning in the community is one of the most important experiences we have at this University. The experiences truly affect the way you look at things. It affects your attitudes and directly reflects on and enhances your success in the academic world.
>
> *Ann Kutney, Nursing Major, University of Scranton*

The term "service-learning" is being echoed in the halls of colleges and universities throughout the nation. Even before students enter these hallowed hallways, service to the community is a concept with which they are becoming increasingly familiar. Many college freshmen have already completed a service-learning requirement in their high schools and will now carry that important experience with them to higher education.

Service, as a reciprocal relationship that contributes to the growth of all people involved, is a popular and important concept in the education of future leaders. Service-learning programs can provide superb learning opportunities for students from a variety of academic disciplines across the university setting and are increasingly being incorporated into areas such as theology and philosophy. The purpose of this book is to detail the concept of service-learning and how this type of program can add to the education of future nurses.

Before one can even begin to look at how service-learning can be incorporated into the nursing curriculum, it is essential to understand what the concept means, along with its historical roots. The interpretation of what service-learning means may differ from one institution to another, from one faculty member to another, and from one student to another. Developing a clear sense of the meaning and components of a solid service-learning program is imperative to the success of any endeavor to incorporate this type of learning into the curriculum. Linking service-learning with traditional liberal arts education and the broader community is an important connection for students. As emphasized by Couto (1982), "These linkages and the emphasis on the institutional context are explicit reminders that behind our institutions and social organizations are people, and that the measure of the worth of these institutions and organizations is how well they service the people within them" (p. xvii).

Chapter One provides an overview of service-learning, historical development of the concept, its many definitions and interpretations, and some basic considerations to examine prior to developing a service-learning program. Highlights of the historical development of service-learning follows.

HISTORICAL OVERVIEW

Before initiating any discussion regarding service-learning, it is important to have a sense of the historical evolution of such programs. Although service-learning programs have been established nationwide in recent years, the idea is not a new one. Rather, the idea of service-learning is one that has been evolving over the past 30 to 40 years.

Essentially, the concept of service-learning in education is a teaching pedagogy that combines several aspects of experiential education, critical thinking, ways of knowing, and civic and personal responsibility. Dewey (1910) advocated this type of learning nearly a century ago. Over the years, these concepts have evolved into what is known today as "education with a community focus" and "education without walls."

In his inaugural address, President Clinton challenged Americans to a "season of service," urging young Americans to give of themselves, to their communities, through actions that will benefit not only the recipient of the service but also the personal and professional growth of the student. "On September 21st, 1993 President Clinton signed into law the landmark national service bill establishing an unprecedented mandate to tackle the nation's pressing challenges through community service" (Pew Health Professions Commission, 1994, p. 5). The president's request led the way for a renewal of the service programs initially started in the 1960s. His request attempted to renew the spirit of Americans everywhere to become engaged, active citizens who care about making a difference in the communities that surround them.

Higher education service-learning programs initially emerged as a result of student community activism in the 1960s and early 1970s. An increased level of consciousness about social problems and issues was developing during that time and the result was the emergence of new community service organizations. According to Couto (1982) "During the student activism of the late sixties, those demanding relevance in education urged student participation in social and political changes and not merely an examination of social and political issues from afar" (p.1). Faculty followed the lead and initiated a dialogue about the connections that could be made between community service activities and the education of students (Mintz & Liu, 1994). Educators knew early on that there had to be a connection between service activities and the education of students if the community programs initiated were to remain viable and meaningful.

One such program is described in detail in the book *Streams of Idealism and Health Care Innovation: An Assessment of Service-Learning and Community Mobilization*, by Richard A. Couto (1982). "In 1969, six medical and nursing students at Vanderbilt University, with financial support from the Josiah C. Macy Foundation, organized the Student Health Coalition" (Couto, 1982, p. 1). This early program focused on educating professional and pre-professional students to address the unmet needs of underserved groups. Comprised primarily of nurses and medical students, this early program paved the way for service-learning programs of the future.

By the late 1970s and early 1980s community service programs were becoming an idea of the past. Those programs that continued on received little attention and no support. Several factors contributed to the decline of these programs. First and foremost, a connection between service and academics had not been clearly established. Lack of this essential connection, along with a reduction in budgets and funding programs for service, meant that the programs that had been initiated could not survive. Finally, other concerns contributing to the downfall of these important programs were lack of a connection to the institution's mission and poor relationships between the institution and surrounding community (Mintz & Liu, 1994). According to Mintz and Liu:

> The problems of this period were aggravated by student attitudes toward community involvement, the larger society's perceptions of students'

commitments and a general societal disengagement with addressing community needs. With an emphasis on gaining material rewards and securing jobs, many students did not associate community service with career success and personal satisfaction. Also, for many students their college experiences were filled with competing priorities and escalating costs. Without institutional support, community service fell low on the priority list. The experiences from the previous two decades offered some important lessons:

1. The community must be a partner in defining its needs.
2. An educational component integrated with the service activity is necessary in order to foster student learning and to enhance the quality of service.
3. Service-learning programs must be aligned into the everyday life of the institution in order to be sustained (Mintz & Liu, 1994, p. 11).

The end of the 1980s saw a renewed interest in service, and the connection established to student learning emerged more clearly. Across the nation, faculty, students, and administrators were now engaged in the development of curricular models that supported service-learning. Now a full-blown movement, service- learning programs have developed across the nation. "Passage of the National Community Service Act of 1990 resulted in hundreds of federally funded service-learning programs across the country" (Mintz & Liu, 1994, p. 11).

Service-learning is a concept that can provide an important dimension to education that will mold and develop important service values in future leaders. Applicable to a variety of educational settings, these programs can offer an important dimension to the preparation of leaders in professional nursing. With an emphasis on critical thinking, nursing students can be exposed to the community setting in a new and different way than what is traditionally expected. Connecting a service experience to educational objectives provides tremendous teaching and learning opportunities. Students can see how their personal interests in nursing can move beyond the traditional care settings and into the communities that surround them.

Reasoning and critical thinking abilities of nursing students can be further refined to ensure the development of community leaders who are positive and committed to problem solving that is meaningful and effective.

Service activities give rise to learning opportunities, and what participants learn further informs their service. Indeed, service-learning is a continuous process of reciprocity that, when implemented with care and expertise, results in high quality service in communities and personal and intellectual development among students (Mintz & Liu, 1994, p. 9).

THE MEANING OF SERVICE-LEARNING

A brief discussion of the meaning of service-learning with faculty and students will reveal a variety of interpretations. Some of the beliefs that are held regarding service-learning are at least partially accurate; others can be problematic to the success of a new program. Therefore, it is important to begin with a clear sense of what a true service-learning program involves and what the concept means. Agreement among nursing faculty regarding the definition of service-learning that is adopted is also a critical starting point prior to the initiation of such programs in the nursing curriculum.

Service-Learning Defined

Robert Sigmon (1979) defined service-learning as an experiential educational approach that is premised on "reciprocal learning." From Sigmon's perspective, learning flows from service activities. Those who are engaged in a service activity and those who are the recipients of service are expected to learn something from the experience. Sigmon emphasized that service-learning occurs only when both the provider and recipients of service benefit from the activities. The definition provided by Sigmon captures the purity and essence of service-learning and allows one to see the relationship between this type of reciprocal learning and course content.

For example, nursing students enrolled in a required major course that covers maternal-child nursing content can become involved in a local "teenage moms" program. Students can provide education regarding child care and age-appropriate vaccines. Students are providing a service to these women and children, while at the same time being sensitized to the special needs of this particular group of people. Learning, therefore, is reciprocal and is further enhanced by reflective discussion in the classroom, a concept discussed in great detail in Chapter Three.

Service programs can vary significantly from one institution to the next. Furco (1996) describes five essential types of service programs. They are:

1. *Volunteerism*;
2. *Community Service*;
3. *Internships*;
4. *Field Education*; and
5. *Service Learning* (Sigmon, 1979).

It is essential to be clear about the type of service program being developed. Sigmon (1979) stated that clear goals must be established for service-learning if we are ever to develop a precise definition: "Each program type is defined by the intended beneficiary of the service activity and its degree of emphasis on service and/or learning" (Furco, 1996, p. 3). Program types can be viewed along a continuum (Furco 1996). Table 1.1 highlights the five program types and the essential differences between each.

As can be seen from the definitions provided in Table 1.1, service-learning is very different than other types of experiential education such as cooperative learning, internships, field practicums, and clinical experiences. The key to a true service-learning program is the "reciprocal relationship." Service is provided to a community based on the community's needs and goals, and the student is provided with a meaningful learning experience that is enhanced through reflection and academic activities. Service-learning links community service and academic study so that each enriches the other. As Hondagneu-Sotelo and Raskoff (1994) emphasized:

> Internships, for example are not always linked directly to the curriculum; field trips may provide one-time snapshots of social groups but do not allow for sustained observations or the development of relationships; in field research courses, the setting provides the context, but not the content, for learning (p. 248).

According to Mintz & Liu (1994):

> Service-learning is a method and philosophy of experiential learning through which participants in community service meet community needs while developing their abilities for critical thinking and group problem-solving, their commitments and values, and the skills they need for effective citizenship. The core elements of service-learning are (1) service activities that help meet community needs that the community finds important, and (2) structured educational components that challenge participants to think critically about and learn from their experiences.

Table 1.1 Differentiating Service Programs as Described by
Furco (1996)

Volunteerism	"Volunteerism is the engagement of students in activities where the primary emphasis is on the service being provided and the primary intended beneficiary is clearly the service recipient" (Furco, p. 4, 1996).
Community Service	"Community service is the engagement of students in activities that primarily focus on the service being provided as well as the benefits the service activities have on the recipients. The students receive some benefits by learning more about how their service makes a difference in the lives of the service recipients" (Furco, p. 4, 1996).
Internships	"Internship programs engage students in service activities primarily for the purpose of providing students with hands-on experiences that enhance their learning or understanding of issues relevant to a particular area of study. Students are the primary intended beneficiary and the focus of the service activity is on student learning" (Furco, p. 4, 1996).
Field Education	"Field education programs provide students with co-curricular service opportunities that are related, but not fully integrated, with their formal academic studies. Students perform the service as a part of a program that is designed primarily to enhance students' understanding of a field of study, while also providing substantial emphasis on the service being provided" (Furco, p. 5, 1996).
Service-Learning	"Service learning programs are distinguished from other approaches to experiential education by their intention to equally benefit the provider and the recipient of the service as well as to ensure equal focus on both the service being provided and the learning that is occurring" (Furco, p. 5, 1996).

The key elements to service-learning can be said to include experiential learning, service that meets identified community needs, and structured educational experiences that include guided reflection that addresses all aspects of the service-learning experience. Capturing the "teachable moments" through reflection and discussion, according to Mintz & Liu (1994) challenges "participants to probe, question, and grapple with their value systems, their preconceptions and stereotypes, and their academic learning" (p. 9). Further, through the reflective process, students can "resolve the tensions that arise during their service experiences, sharpen their ability to reason, to think critically, and to be more effective and committed problem solvers" (Mintz & Liu, p. 9).

SERVICE AS AN INSTRUMENT OF EDUCATION

Service-learning programs can only be an instrument of education when they are connected to an academic learning experience. Participants must be engaged in organized community service that will provide short- and long-term benefits to the community being served. Additionally, structured opportunities to reflect on the actual experience, discuss, and learn from what transpired must be included in a true service-learning program. As Mintz and Liu (1994) emphasized, service-learning programs should

> foster collaboration both within the institution and between the institution and the community. In this capacity, the resources of the institution contribute to the welfare of the community, and the community is a contributing partner in education. Programs should combine the talents and resources of faculty, students, administrators, community based agencies, and individual community members in order to achieve the objectives of service-learning (p. 10).

The service-learning experience must be relevant to and enhance the student's academic curriculum. As Bringle and Hatcher (1996) noted:

> We view service learning as a credit-bearing educational experience in which students participate in an organized service activity that meets identified community needs and reflects on the service activity in such a way as to gain further understanding of course content, a broader appreciation of the discipline, and an enhanced sense of civic responsibility (p. 222).

Students will make the connection between academics and service early on as well, if the program is well grounded and faculty are prepared to make connections between the service activity and the theory. As one University of Scranton student noted: "Service-learning is the opportunity to bring together what you learn in the classroom and what you get from going to a Jesuit University in the community. Learning occurs through providing a service to your community". Table 1.2 offers additional examples of students' perceptions of service-learning and how their experiences have contributed to their personal and professional growth.

Course connected service-learning experiences offer students the most opportunity for obtaining an educational experience that truly reflects the reciprocal relationship expected. With some planning and resources, faculty can incorporate service-learning as a requirement for a specific course. Allocating a percentage of the course grade for assignments such as journaling activity, reflection papers, and in-class discussion of service activities helps to connect the service experience with academic learning. Incorporating service-learning into a specific nursing course works well, since most nursing content already has a service component that can be connected to a community setting. For example, in an introductory nursing course, a service-learning experience can be designed to meet an identified community need while at the same time providing freshman nursing majors with some sense of what the profession involves. Table 1.3 offers some points for students to consider and will help faculty interested in initiating a service-learning requirement.

Other options for the incorporation of service-learning into the curriculum include a separate service-learning course or a service requirement outside the classroom setting. The last two options can be valuable experiences for student learning. However, they may lack the close supervision and connection to an academic field that is provided when the service-learning occurs as a component of a required course. Incorporation of service-learning in the curriculum is also addressed in Chapter Two.

If your university has an office specifically designed to address community service, it may be helpful to begin to develop a service-learning component in the nursing major with the help of individuals from this office. Many colleges and universities already have these services available, and they can provide a place to begin. These offices are generally skilled in providing up-to-date information on community needs and can act as liaisons with agency personnel. Some examples of service-learning experiences that may be relevant to students in nursing and other majors include working with the learning disabled in school settings; developing

Table 1.2 Student Reflections Regarding Service-Learning

"My service learning hours were completed at the Boys and Girls Club. Here I helped the children with their homework, and played games and sports. I realized that these children come from very diverse backgrounds and many have unstable family lives. This was evident by their lack of discipline and their need for constant attention. I tried my best to keep up with their demanding needs but realized that I could not please everyone. This is where my decision making and authoritative skills were refined. I had to constantly keep thinking of solutions to little problems. There were also times when the children would get bored and complain that there was nothing to do. This is when my problem-solving skills became effective, and I needed to think of something fun to keep them occupied."

"There were aspects of the service-learning experience that were not so enjoyable. It hurt to see children come in day after day looking so dirty, sometimes I just wanted to give them a bath. I also found it hard to hear some children talk about how they did not want to go home because they did not like it there. It hurt me to see so many children with a poor family life and this came as a wake up call, because I realized how lucky I am to have a loving family who is always there for me."

"Before my service-learning experience I hardly considered the elderly or dying as part of the community. It is the people of my generation that are usually the focus of my thought processes. By spending time with the elderly, those in poor health and with the dying, I think my awareness is raised a bit. And every week when I spend a few hours with them I am exposed to the perspective of the people I rarely consider."

"I learned many things about myself through my service experience this spring. Primarily, I was able to develop some characteristics of my personality that I was not aware of before hand. I would normally categorize myself as a shy, reserved person. At the Veteran's Center, however, I found a completely different side of myself; I notice that I could be an outgoing individual. I would like to find a balance for myself. One of the most important things I have learned at the Vet Center is that when you can communicate effectively with other people, you can learn so much about others and about yourself."

"I feel that learning in the community impacts my academic life here at the University. While I was volunteering I learned more about what kind of person I am and more about others. I don't think that I realized this as much before I started volunteering. This has also affected my academic life. I now think about other things in life besides my studies, which has resulted in less

Table 1.2 *(continued)*

stress. I am receiving higher grades now which could be related to my overall feeling of well-being. I believe that only good things come out of service-learning. Through this work both the students and the recipient benefit."

"I learned that the community needs a lot of help. I never realized how many single-parent families there are and the effect this has on the children. Many of the children lack a male and female role model, or lack a role model as a whole."

"I really feel that this experience helped me in more ways than I could even begin to count. It not only made me aware of the everyday functions of a hospital, it made me realize that someday I will be in charge and I need to strive to be the best nurse I possibly can be."

recreational programs in prison settings; assisting in a senior citizen center; participating in peer education programs for HIV/AIDS; becoming a hospice volunteer; or helping with after-school programs, such as those offered by the Boys and Girls Club of America.

The opportunities for service-learning connected to an academic course requirement are endless and limited only by one's creativity and imagination. In the nursing major, for example, the required community nursing course can be used to do a needs assessment on the surrounding community. The data gathered can then be used to develop service-learning experiences for students that are connected to academics, while once again meeting identified community needs (See Appendix G).

Adequate preparation in terms of establishing contacts and setting up appropriate placements is also essential. Students must have some basic preparation prior to being sent out into a community agency. Table 1.4 offers some guidelines for students as they plan their service-learning experience. Table 1.5 highlights some of the rights and responsibilities of students in service-learning programs.

THE BENEFITS OF SERVICE-LEARNING

The benefits of a service-learning program for those just beginning can only be imagined. Specific examples of the important educational

Table 1.3 Essential Steps for Students: Planning the Service-Learning Experience

PRIOR TO COMMITTING TO A SPECIFIC SERVICE LEARNING EXPERIENCE CONSIDER THE FOLLOWING:

1. What is your schedule? What days and hours are best for you to be available to complete your service-learning hours?

2. How will you travel to your assigned agency? Do you need transportation or is the agency within safe walking distance?

3. Are you able to commit to the number of hours and the scheduled times required by the particular agency?

4. Will you be able to follow through with your commitment to the agency and complete the required hours?

5. Is your schedule flexible enough to meet the needs of the agency?

6. Review the list of agencies offering community service opportunities. Do any of them match your course objectives and the issues with which you would like to work? Discuss your options with your course faculty member.

7. Select one agency and call the contact person. Be persistent; sometimes, staff are difficult to reach. Once you have made contact, tell them where you attend school and explain the nature of your service-learning assignment. Be sure to ask any questions that you have.

8. Set up a time to visit the agency, become oriented and discuss your roles and responsibilities with the agency preceptor.

9. Schedule your times at the agency

10. Be punctual and reliable in your service.

opportunities that can emerge in a service-learning experience are discussed throughout this book. The combination of service with reflective teaching will offer all those participating in a service program the opportunity to grow personally and professionally.

In terms of nursing education, it is expected that students will complete essential content in such areas as medical-surgical, obstetrics, pediatrics, and mental health nursing. The addition of a service-learning component to any of these areas provides the nursing student with new opportunities not offered in any other way. As nursing care moves from the acute care setting to the community, these service experiences become even more

Table 1.4 Rights and Responsibilities of Students Engaged in Service-Learning Experiences

---

WHAT THE AGENCY EXPECTS FROM THE STUDENT
- Dependability and reliability in fulfilling hours
- An honest assessment of your abilities, interest and skills
- Active participation in the agency orientation program
- Professional behavior, including observance of any dress code and respect for confidentiality
- Willingness to follow policies and procedures of the agency
- Advanced notice (24 hours) if you expect to be absent from your planned service

WHAT YOU CAN EXPECT FROM THE AGENCY
- An orientation to the site and training for the expected service
- Guidance, direction, and input from agency personnel
- Respect from others serving in the community agency
- An opportunity to make suggestions, get feedback, and develop a sense of being an integral part of the program
- An evaluation of your efforts at the end of the experience
- Appreciation for your efforts in serving the community

KEEP THE FOLLOWING POINTS IN MIND:
- Know who is in charge. Be sure you have their name and phone number in case you need to contact them
- Get to know the area around the community site
- Know the rules
- Let a roommate or friend know your schedule
- Keep up with what is going on in the agency
- Listen to your instincts in questionable situations

---

valuable. For example, in a course covering illnesses primarily affecting women, such as breast cancer, a valuable service-learning experience might be to have students offer programs in self-breast examination and early detection. Taking this information to low-income housing neighborhoods where these individuals might not otherwise have access to prevention information takes the content into the community, to an area with an identified need. Students can then learn, through reflection in the classroom setting, a great deal about themselves, their belief systems, and the needs of the communities that surround them.

Table 1.5 Faculty Guide : Steps to Integrating Service-Learning

---

BEFORE THE SEMESTER BEGINS

1. Confer with resource persons available on your campus. These might include other colleagues experienced in service-learning and staff available in offices dealing directly with community service.

2. Determine what agencies will be used for service-learning experiences related to your course.

3. Develop the syllabus and incorporate service-learning as a component of the course assignments. Each faculty person will be unique in the design of their own syllabus. Following are some suggestions for inclusion in a course that is integrating service-learning:
  • Service-learning requirement is included in the course description
  • Definition of service-learning and its connection to course content
  • Specific objectives that address outcomes for service-learning
  • Designated times for group reflection (mid semester/end of semester)
  • 15 hours required for service
  • Written assignments (reaction papers, dialogue journals, etc)
  • Allocation of points/credit toward final course grade

DURING THE FIRST TWO WEEKS OF THE SEMESTER

1. Discuss the service-learning component of the course with students and how it relates to their academic work and learning experiences.

2. Work with students as they select agencies in which they will complete their service-learning requirements.

  If you have decided that students in your course should have a service experience in one or two specific agencies (because of relationship to course objectives/content) then it is important for you to initiate contact with that agency prior to the beginning of the semester, to determine their needs and to begin to establish a "partnership" with them for continued service-learning experiences for students in your particular course. If you are allowing students to decide their service experience for themselves, you will need to give them some guidance and feedback on the choices they make.

  It is essential that students be oriented to the agencies with which they will be working. The community agency usually assumes this responsibility. However, it is important for the faculty member to take some time in class to review with students their responsibilities as members of the University community as they begin their service-learning experiences. Issues of communication, appropriate dress, interpersonal relations with agency personnel and those being served, and accountability for fulfilling the service contract should be reviewed with students prior to beginning the service. Faculty need to spell out, very carefully, the goals and objectives of the experience and how it relates to course content.

Table 1.5 *(continued)*

THROUGHOUT THE SEMESTER

1. Students should complete the required hours for the service-learning experience.

2. Reflection activities such as class discussion and journal writing take place and are correlated to class learning.

3. At mid-semester, evaluate how the service-learning experience is working for students.

END OF SEMESTER

1. Students complete all course requirements for the service-learning experience.

2. Completed assignments and required paperwork related to the service learning experience are handed in.

3. Final reflection takes place.

4. Evaluate the service-learning experience with students, agency personnel, and faculty.

METHODS OF EVALUATION

There are many ways to evaluate how the service-learning experience is progressing within your course and how it is affecting student learning. How you evaluate the experience will depend on your course objectives and the degree to which the service is integrated into your course. It is very important that student assignments allow for connections to be made between course content and service in the community. This will demonstrate the educational value you place on the service-learning experience. The number of hours required (10, 15, 20) will also have an impact on what is learned and how you and the student can evaluate the experience.

SOME POSSIBLE EVALUATION STRATEGIES

- Ongoing reading of and commenting on student journals
- Class reflection times
- Reaction papers, case studies, or projects
- Class presentations
- Observation/participation at service sites
- Agency evaluation of student service
- Faculty and student evaluation of the overall experience

Service-learning provides valuable experiences when it is connected to the course content and shows the student how the theory and practice flow beyond the walls of the university and hospital setting and into the community. These opportunities allow students to meet new people and be exposed to new ideas. Connections are established between academics and the community at large. Finally, the experiences can build character, increase awareness of career possibilities, and enhance leadership skills. Moving beyond traditional healthcare settings and working with people from different backgrounds challenges the students' personal belief and value systems, and allows them to grow intellectually. Questions may be raised about inequality and injustice in terms of healthcare access for all people. Through structured reflection, the student learns and grows from these experiences.

It is expected that the service-learning experience will be a positive one; however, as with all experiences, there will always be exposure to negative aspects in a particular setting. Both the positive and negative aspects of the experience must be drawn into the reflective process to allow the student to learn and grow from the opportunity that has been provided. Some of the possible outcomes that may result from the service-learning experience include: an opportunity to add enrichment to a required course that might not have been possible by simply participating in a classroom setting; identification of areas of interest for future career development; enhancement of leadership skills; improved self-awareness; and establishing an understanding and concern for social problems that exist in one's community and awareness of one's responsibility to the community. A true service-learning experience that has been well focused with a strong reflective component can prepare the way for continued citizenship throughout life. Students develop an acute awareness of the problems that exist in their immediate geographical community and see how they can be active in making meaningful changes.

INITIATING A SERVICE-LEARNING PROGRAM

Initiating a service-learning program is not without difficulties. Many of the issues that can present as problems are discussed in Chapter four of this book. A commitment to this type of educational experience will provide a foundation to deal with both the promises and pitfalls that develop along the way. Coordination and support of the program begin with faculty but must also come from administration. Further, there must be a connection to the mission of the university.

Faculty leadership is essential to the success of a service-learning program. "With such leadership, service can become an integral part of the learning experience. Without it, service is reduced to charity, and learning happens only accidentally" (Wills, 1992, p. 36). Faculty are the key to the long-term commitment to public service and to meaningful learning within a community.

Being clear about what service-learning means in relationship to the program and overall mission of the college or university is a starting point. Faculty commitment and leadership will provide the foundations for a successful program.

SUMMARY

This chapter examined the meaning of service-learning and its historical roots. From the early 1960s to the present-day concept, service-learning has always been a meaningful and important component of the educational experience. The development of service-learning is grounded in the reciprocal learning that occurs between the individual providing the service and those being served. Programs that have strong faculty leadership, clear methods of identifying community needs, and a connection to the mission of the academic setting can flourish and become an integral part of the student's learning experience. The success of any service-learning program will be determined by clear objectives and faculty commitment. For additional references related to developing a service-learning program, please refer to Appendix A.

REFERENCES

Bringle, R. G., & Hatcher, J. A. (1996). Implementing service learning in higher education. *Journal of Higher Education, 67*(2), 222–239.

Couto, R. A. (1982). *Streams of idealism and health care innovation: An assessment of service-learning and community mobilization.* New York: Teachers College Press.

Dewey, J. (1910). *How we think.* New York: D.C.

Furco, A. (1996). "Service-Learning: A balanced approach to experiential education." In *Expanding Boundaries: Service and Learning*, 2–5. Washington, DC: Corporation for National Service.

Hondagneu-Sotelo, P., & Raskoff, S. (1994). Community service-learning: Promises and problems. *Teaching Sociology, 22*, 248–254.

Honnet, E. P., & Poulsen, S. J.(1994). Principles of good practice for combining service and learning. *Wingspread Special Report*. Raciue, Wisconsin: The Johnson Foundation, Inc.

Mintz, S., & Liu, G. (1994). Service-learning: An overview. In *Health Professions Schools in Service to the Nation Workshop Guide*, 9–11.

The Pew Health Professions Commission in Partnership with The Bureau of Health Professions, U.S. Public Health Service and The Corporation for National and Community Service, (1994). *Health Professions Schools in Service to the Nation Workshop Guide*, 1–61.

Sigmon, Robert L. (1979). Service-learning: Three principles. *Synergist, 8*(1), 9–11.

Wills, R. L. (1992). Service on campus and in the curriculum. *Education Record*, Vol 73 Issue 2, 32–36.

CHAPTER 2

Integrating Service-Learning into the Curriculum

Patricia Harrington, Ed.D, R.N.

> I believe that we have affected a population that some
> people don't even think exists.
>
> —*Eileen Healey, Nursing Student, HIV Outreach*

Incorporating service-learning into the nursing curriculum is a challenging yet manageable task. The challenge that presents itself is related to the fact that most nursing curricula are "credit-heavy." In many programs, half of the nursing credits are for clinical experiences which, very often, are 3 hours for one credit. Nursing students usually spend between 10 and 20 hours per week in a clinical setting giving direct care to patients. Given this time commitment, finding room to fit service into the students' schedule can be difficult. However, even with their very full schedules, most students believe service experiences are well worth the time. Hales (1997) agrees and reminds us that nursing philosophy is based on service to others, and that the care of vulnerable groups has long been entrusted to nurses. Participating in service-learning allows students to live the philosophy of nursing while learning from others in the community about the essence of caring for all people. This chapter will address the necessary steps for incorporating service-learning in the nursing curriculum. Strategies for a successful program are discussed, along with some suggestions for heading off problems before they begin.

ESSENTIAL COMPONENTS FOR SUCCESSFUL SERVICE-LEARNING PROGRAMS

There are a number of necessary components for successful implementation of a service-learning program. These curricular components include student motivation, faculty interest, timing, content, and supervision. Each required component is discussed in detail in this chapter.

Certainly, the value of hands-on experience has always been recognized as essential to learning the art and science of nursing. As noted in the introduction, the amount of clinical time required for nursing courses can hinder both student and faculty willingness to participate in a service-learning experience. Further, the timing of service experiences must fit around required clinical hours, and this may limit the options available to students. With limited options, students may settle for experiences that fit their schedule, rather than selecting an experience that is meaningful to them and their academic work.

Faculty must play a key role in guiding the selection of service-learning activities for students. Very often, however, faculty are limited by time constraints and may also be uncomfortable with unsupervised service activities. In terms of these unsupervised service activities, consideration must be given to issues of accountability, student performance, and safety. Comprehensive planning for service-learning experiences is vital for success. A detailed discussion of the key components for a successful service-learning program follows.

Student Motivation

Student motivation is one key component that is critical to the development of a service-learning program. One way to engage students and motivate them to develop an interest in service is to introduce them to service-learning in required freshman nursing courses. If there are no required nursing courses in the freshman level of the program, perhaps an interdisciplinary course or separate service-learning course can be developed (See Appendices F and G for examples of course integration of service-learning).

Before service-learning was incorporated into the first required nursing course, freshman nursing majors were repeatedly requesting "clinical experiences" earlier in the program. Clearly, a clinical experience at that point would not have been appropriate for a variety of reasons. Without a sound foundation in the sciences and no basic clinical skills, it would be foolish to even consider this option. With the incorporation of service-learning, students can select a service site that is of interest to them and that has a connection to the practice of professional nursing. This opportunity allows the student to experience "clinical" from a different perspective. Students are provided with a view of the nurse's role and at the same time have some sense that they have experienced one aspect of hands-on nursing.

For example, one freshman nursing major with little experience around children identified her own need to increase her comfort level with children before the junior-year pediatric rotation. She chose a day-care center as her service-learning site and was able to increase her comfort level with preschoolers long before the pediatric course. In most cases, students choose areas they have some familiarity with, which helps in terms of comfort level and increases their motivation to participate.

Interestingly, many freshmen chose hospital sites for their service-learning experience, while junior and senior nursing majors tended to select community sites. The seniors reported that by junior year they had enough clinical and needed a break from the fast-paced hospital setting. This emphasizes further how life experience can change what is important and meaningful to all people. Senior nursing majors also bring more confidence and maturity to the experience which adds to their community interest.

When first presented with the service-learning requirement, students participate because they are externally motivated. Service-learning is a course requirement that must be completed in order to successfully achieve course objectives. Many students will remain externally motivated, and while they truly enjoy the service experience, they participate only because it is required. Other students will internalize the commitment to service and complete additional hours over and above the requirements of a particular course. This, of course, is the ideal situation, and one of the main objectives associated with a service-learning program.

The internalization of service as a lifelong experience can occur early in a course of study or at almost any time during the student's education. Some freshman nursing majors continued to serve in the community agency with which they fulfilled their course requirement during the summer months. Letters from community partners attest to this, and help to validate the positive nature of the service-learning experience. In reflection groups, students share the profound commitments they have developed, and their enthusiasm for their area of service can be contagious. Faculty can continue to motivate students through appropriate feedback on journals and during reflection sessions. One can see there are many avenues to developing and maintaining student motivation for service-learning. Tapping into a variety of motivational strategies works best in most situations.

Motivation can dwindle when student expectations of the service experience are not met, or when their relationship with the agency partner is not working out. Sometimes expectations are diminished because of personality conflicts, or perhaps the students might find themselves in a service-learning setting that simply is not interesting to them. Regular communication through journals, checking in with agencies where students are assigned, and reflective sessions will alert faculty to problems that may be easily resolved. Students should be encouraged to share and evaluate service-learning experiences openly and honestly with their faculty member. At times, it may be beneficial to permit students to change to another site when their expectations are not being met. Allowing students to change their service site helps to avoid reinforcement of negative stereotypes that can develop. For instance, working in a nursing home may reinforce a student's belief that all elderly people are weak and frail. Instead, changing the site to a center for active elderly may help to change or avoid the negative attitude.

Faculty Interest

Faculty interest is central for successful integration of service-learning (Bringle & Hatcher, 1996; Stanton, 1991; Wills, 1992). Nursing faculty play a major role in the success of the program. While direct supervision is not required, students do need feedback and guidance. Ideally, the faculty teaching the course in which service-learning is required should read student journals, run reflection sessions, and interact with the service agencies. Some faculty may even choose to become directly involved in service activities. These activities require extra work on the part of faculty and the time constraints of agendas filled with research requirements can be discouraging to faculty and prevent involvement in service-learning. Often, faculty agree that service-learning programs are important . . . just not for their courses.

The content for most nursing courses is highly prescribed and intense; making the addition of a service requirement even more burdensome in the eyes of some faculty and students. Institutional support can provide a graduate assistant or service-learning liaison to assist faculty with journals, reflection sessions, and agency relationships in an effort to alleviate some of the time- intensive work. Other incentives for faculty include extra credit or release time for incorporating service-learning into a required course. Providing financial support to attend conferences and visit institutions with service-learning models further supports the introduction of the teaching pedagogy into the nursing curriculum.

Institutional requirements for faculty participation in service are usually very broad. This may present yet another stumbling block for faculty with regard to service-learning. While the majority of universities stress that service is an important part of the faculty role, the emphasis for promotion is on faculty research activities. Zlotkowski (1996) laments that although faculty are interested in linking education and service, they are not incorporating a commitment to service in their own professional lives.

Connecting service-learning activities with teaching and research interests of faculty is an excellent way to maximize experiences for the students and create enthusiasm for service-learning among faculty. Allowing and encouraging faculty to share their service, teaching, and research interests with students can be most fruitful for the development of a meaningful and effective service-learning agenda. Chapter Five offers the reader examples of successful programs initiated in the service-learning program described in this text.

Timing

Helping students find the time to fit service requirements into their busy schedules is also very important. A 15-hour semester requirement seems like a lot on the first day of class when students are preoccupied with intensive course requirements that are being presented. In the program described in this text, the faculty were initially concerned that the addition of such a requirement would be too overwhelming for the students given the workload already required. This led to a discussion about reducing the service-learning requirement for junior nursing majors and perhaps increasing hours for freshman and sophomore students. Much to everyone's surprise, in the final course evaluation, most students reported that the service requirement worked well, and they felt it was an important part of the course. Only a few students suggested that it be dropped as a requirement.

Certainly, when an individual student experiences difficulty in managing academic and service responsibilities, faculty need to be flexible with the service requirements. For example, one student, a mother of three small children, was allowed to complete her service hours in the long-term care setting where she worked. Her service hours were in addition to her work hours, but the convenience of the service site made the requirement more manageable in this instance. Each time the service-learning requirement is implemented, new situations and difficulties may emerge. Most are easily resolved with some flexibility, patience, and creativity.

Offering students a variety of choices in both the type of service agency they are assigned to and the hours in which they can complete the service helps them to match their interests and needs with those of the agency. Some students may only be able to commit to service on the weekends or evenings. For these students, a hospital setting or an after-school center may be most appealing. For others, a one or two full-day service opportunity may be more realistic. Habitat for Humanity is a good choice when students need a large number of hours in a few days. Other choices include one-day campus service events. For example, at the University of Scranton, a program for the mentally and physically challenged in the Scranton community is held each semester. The program, known as "Hand-in-Hand", provides students with the opportunity to work with one or two individuals, taking them through carnival events for one day. The American Red Cross is another excellent community site offering nursing students a variety of service opportunities. Most local chapters provide the training for programs, including:

1) Blood Services, taking health histories and checking hemoglobin levels at local blood drives;
2) HIV instructors, providing their peers and high school students with HIV-prevention information;
3) Disaster Nursing, preparing for future community emergencies; and
4) Water Safety and CPR instructors.

Providing choices with regard to time and type of service site enables the faculty to maximize the benefits of service-learning. Students can easily select a schedule and a site they are interested in when variety and flexibility are part of a service-learning program.

Content

Ideally, the service experiences should be related to the course content. In some instances, however, this may not be possible. It is acceptable to identify community needs and then place students in agencies even if the service is not directly connected to the academic course work. Students may select an after-school club working with pre-teens in a sports program in their freshman or sophomore course and plan to continue this in their junior year.

How will these experiences relate to content in an adult medical-surgical or psychiatric nursing course? Actually, any service activity can complement the nursing curriculum. An important objective of all clinical nursing courses, regardless of the setting, is the development of therapeutic communication skills. All students, regardless of their service setting, are able to develop or improve upon these skills. In fact, when asked to reflect on the value of their experiences, students frequently identified the opportunity to utilize therapeutic communication skills as an important benefit of their service experiences.

There is also a much broader benefit to service-learning that enhances any course content. That benefit is the overall development of the student from an observer to a change agent. Buchen (1995) proposed that the effect of service-learning on the student is a "transfusion" that stimulates academic growth. He described six developmental stages that occur in the student from "needing to be needed, to know more and understand why" to "knowing what can be changed" and actually, "knowing how to change it" (p. 67). As students participate in service projects, they learn more about "others" than they could possibly learn from books. According to Buchen, they are able to blend what they learn from service in the community with the academic content they learn in class. They begin, in the freshman year, feeling "good about helping others," and move to intervening with community partners in the senior year with the goal to "improve the health of a neighborhood."

Through group reflection and journal writing, students identify aspects of their service-learning experiences that connect to course content. For example, while one group of students worked with children, the majority of the class served adults in hospice, long-term care, and the emergency room. Through reflection sessions with the entire class, students' experiences were shared and they learned from each other. Several students enrolled in hospice training between semesters after learning about their peers' experiences during reflection sessions. In the subsequent semester, they again chose hospice as their service site. Connecting the content and the service, through feedback in journals and reflection sessions, enables the student to move from needing to help others to being able to make a difference. Certainly there is the potential that through service-learning students will make important career decisions. Learning about an area of interest or growing in a new area contributes to the education of the students and adds to the information they gather to help them make choices about their lives and their careers.

Supervision

Supervision of students in service-learning experiences is a key component to the overall success of a program. One of the drawbacks to community-based service is the difficulty in supervising students at a variety of sites. Few agencies can accommodate groups of students, and service activities can occur at a variety of hours, 7 days a week. Faculty may object to or have legitimate concerns regarding unsupervised service-learning experiences.

Specific criteria should guide student placement in agencies and alleviate some of the concerns associated with unsupervised service-learning activities. Many agencies have extensive criteria and training programs for the students who wish to serve as volunteers. These programs are helpful in terms of assuring that students are adequately prepared for the service experience. Placing students in agencies where faculty provide service is another way to enhance communication about student performance. In the absence of faculty presence, community partners who work with students play an important role in supervision and evaluation of the students' performance.

Journal entries after each service experience can also give faculty information regarding the service experience and facilitate the necessary supervision. Students should be encouraged to report any unusual events immediately to the faculty member. Instances of abuse or neglect, for example, would require immediate action. The student's relationship with the faculty member is crucial here. One example is an instance where a student observed a new employee in a long-term care facility handling a patient in a rough manner during care. The student reported the incident to the faculty member who, in turn, notified the agency and the university. The agency followed up on the incident and counseled the employee appropriately. In another situation, two students, serving in the emergency room of a local hospital, observed the care of a victim of an automobile accident who did not survive. They reported the event in class the next day and were encouraged to verbalize their feelings and express any fears that they experienced. These examples emphasize the importance of open communication between faculty and students.

Supervision is a challenging aspect of service-learning. Support from the institution is needed in the form of reassigned hours or financial compensation for faculty. Financial support for faculty to direct service-learning programs or the support of graduate assistants is sometimes available through grant funding. Both private and governmental sources should be explored. With sufficient time to coordinate community placements, supervise students, and evaluate the experience for all participants—students, community agencies, and the people served—faculty can develop effective programs that will enhance student learning and fulfill the university's service mission in the community.

OPTIONS FOR INCORPORATING SERVICE-LEARNING

There are a variety of ways to incorporate service-learning into the curriculum. Enos and Troppe (1996) describe ten methods including:

1) A fourth- credit option;
2) Introductory service-learning courses;
3) Leadership courses;
4) A limited course component;
5) An extensive course requirement;
6) Part of the core curriculum;
7) A graduation requirement;
8) A capstone project;
9) A research project; and
10) An internship.

The various options described by Enos and Troppe (1996) allow faculty to match the method with the course and with the discipline. The "Fourth Credit Option" offers students the opportunity to gain academic credit for their service activities. One credit is added to the course for students choosing the service option. It is helpful for students who can use the extra credits; however, it may not be needed by many nursing majors, as most nursing curricula have few elective course or credit options.

Introductory service-learning courses usually include a significant number of service hours, possibly 30 or more per semester (Enos & Troppe, 1996). Some are interdisciplinary, with a wide variety of service options, and may not fit into the nursing curriculum. For students in majors that have elective course options, an introductory service-learning course in freshman year can help them to identify a service site of interest to them. In subsequent semesters, the students can further explore the community's needs and develop and implement interventions that make a difference for the people served. Starting with extensive hours provides an opportunity to become familiar with the agency's mission and the community's needs, enabling students to plan future service projects.

Service-learning as community leadership is an attractive opportunity for many students, especially those whose majors focus on social issues. Enos & Troppe (1996) site examples of this type of service course, several of which focus on a series of experiences that build leadership skills in students over several semesters. Other courses tailor experiences to give students a general view of community activism related to the students' area of study.

Experiences for nursing majors can be designed to include leadership experiences as they progress through their program. At the University of Scranton, the senior community health course offered several leadership options for students (See Appendix G). One group of students, who were HIV peer educators (on campus) for their sophomore and junior service hours, developed an HIV community outreach project for disadvantaged women and children in cooperation with the American Red Cross. The students incorporated a pre- and post-test assessment and presented their findings at a national service-learning conference. The HIV Women's Outreach program is discussed in detail in Chapter Five, as an example of a successful community partnership.

Service-learning can also be incorporated as a "limited component of the course." In nursing, there are already extensive clinical requirements (210–250 hours per semester); therefore, utilizing service-learning as a "limited component of the course" worked well for faculty in the early development and integration of service-learning into the curriculum. This method focuses on students participating in 15 hours of service (for the semester), and reflecting on the experience as it relates to the course, rather than focusing on community outcomes (Enos and Troppe, 1996). Using service-learning as a limited component of the course was effective for the freshman and sophomore courses. For the two junior semesters, in which students had 15 hours per week of clinical, dedicating even 15 service hours during the semester was difficult. Service-learning requirements included keeping a dialogue journal, participating in classroom reflection sessions, and submitting a reaction paper analyzing the experience and how it related to the students' personal and academic life. Enos and Troppe (1996) warn that limited service requirements may reinforce negative beliefs about vulnerable populations. Students will sometimes share these negative beliefs in journals and in reflection. It is helpful for the reflection leader (if it is someone other than the faculty member) to read the journals and ask students to share important experiences in order to help dispel stereotypes that other students may have.

Requiring service-learning as an extensive course requirement compels faculty to carefully structure the experiences and connect them to the course work. In universities where service is an extensive course requirement, specific criteria are followed that include relating the course theory and the service, soliciting evaluations from the recipients of the service, and providing opportunities for students to learn from the service activities of their peers (Enos & Troppe, 1996).

The use of service-learning as an "extensive component of the course" may be appropriate for senior community and leadership experiences. Students develop a sense of what the community needs by their senior year through their clinical experiences, service activities, and research. Trusting relationships with both the agency partners and the people who are served have been established at this point in the students' education. Students are ready, in most cases, to implement a community service project that can be a significant contribution to those served.

The next step for the program described in this text is to expand service-learning in the senior-year community health course where students can enhance their clinical experiences with service-learning activities. One option may include the administration of a health survey to residents of a low-income housing development. Through service-learning, the students would be introduced to the community and, based on the results of the survey, develop a health promotion project that they can implement during required clinical hours. During the same semester, students enrolled in nursing research, may choose to design their research project to examine some aspect of their service project. The capstone experience can be the presentation of a poster addressing the service and research projects conducted.

Requiring service-learning as part of the core curriculum extends the opportunity to more students (Enos & Troppe, 1996). For nursing majors, participating in service-learning in a humanities course would enhance the connection between the arts and scientific nursing knowledge. Darbyshire

(1994) makes this connection through the study of literature about home-lessness and AIDS where nursing students view the experience of illness from the patients' perspective. Stanton (1991) agrees that incorporating service-learning into study of the humanities will enhance the develop-ment of civic responsibility in students. In universities where service-learning opportunities are offered in the humanities, students have wider opportunities to explore service in different ways. Opportunities for sum-mer courses in other countries combined with service projects, give stu-dents a global perspective of the need for service and the experiences of others. In addition, nursing majors often find it easier to fit a summer course into their schedules.

Requiring service for graduation can be an administrative challenge; however, it does emphasize the importance of service to the student (Enos & Troppe, 1996). At the University of Scranton, community service is a requirement for all students enrolled in one division, known as the J. A. Panuska College of Professional Studies. Several departments in the divi-sion, including nursing, have incorporated the service requirement into existing courses. Monitoring service activities that are within courses, rather than those that occur separate from an academic course, is much more manageable as well as meaningful. By requiring service-learning as a component of several courses, we can assist the students in building on earlier service experiences and on the shared experiences of other students.

Incorporation of service-learning as a capstone or a research project can provide a very meaningful experience for students. In this way, students can identify and critically analyze community needs over several semes-ters, develop research questions, and conduct pilot studies with results that will contribute to the community's strategy for change. The next step is to encourage faculty to engage in research that serves the community and connects the research project to service-learning.

Finally, incorporating service-learning through an internship is another possibility to consider. Enos & Troppe (1996) advised that the service-learning aspect of the internship should be guided reflection and develop-ment of a commitment to community service, in addition to the traditional purposes of internships, such as clarification of career goals for students. Porter and Schwartz (1993) described a service-learning model used in a sociology course where they combined a traditional classroom course, "The Sociology of AIDS," with an internship. Students in the course served at HIV/AIDS agencies for 4 hours per week, and were involved in actual service activities. Class assignments that were based on the service included a term paper analyzing an issue they faced in the agency, along with a weekly journal about their service and their reaction to lectures and guest speakers. Even though the hours were extensive, the students rated their experiences highly. They reported that service experiences were essential to understanding sociological theories.

Clark, Spence, and Sheehan (1987) utilized a service-learning model in a course for health professionals about health and aging. Using an interdisciplinary framework, they brought together students from nursing, medicine, counseling, pharmacy, nutrition, and dental hygiene to deliver health promotion workshops to elderly in community sites. The focus of the course was the service experience with weekly seminars designed to prepare the students for their work and to give them opportunities to report on the health promotion workshops. Strategies were developed to enhance the interdisciplinary approach. Capstone preceptorships are required in many nursing programs and could be easily converted into a service-learning focus with the addition of reflection and sharing of service experiences in class.

STRUCTURING THE SERVICE EXPERIENCE

The process of incorporating service-learning takes planning, perseverance, attention to detail, and revisions based on ongoing evaluation. Development of strong community partnerships is an essential ingredient to a successful program. In planning the service-learning program at the University of Scranton, we identified community agencies who focused on health promotion and restoration and who worked with our students in the past. The Office of Collegiate Volunteers was active in placing students in community service sites, and relationships with a wide variety of agencies were already established.

Examination of nursing student service over 5 years prior to the implementation of the service-learning program revealed that many had regularly engaged in service to the community. Four agencies were targeted for structured experiences, and included: 1) The American Red Cross; 2) The Jewish Home for Elderly; 3) The Boys and Girls Club; and 4)The VNA Hospice. Representatives from each agency were invited to serve on a Service-Learning Advisory Board. At the beginning of each semester, students were given a list of service options that included four targeted agencies along with a variety of other community groups. In order to maintain strong student motivation, they were not limited in their choices.

Service-learning was piloted in a freshman nursing course for the first time in the spring of 1995. Although at that time the service-learning experience was optional, 95% of the class chose the assignment (See Appendix F for a sample program design). Results were positive and the next year, it was a course requirement for freshman. Each subsequent year, the service-learning requirement was incorporated into at least one course per year (See Appendix E for program planning). The graduates of 1998 were the first class that participated in service-learning throughout their nursing education. They played an important role in planning, implementing, and revising the current service-learning program.

The most effective approaches to service-learning are those that are based on course objectives and that assist students to understand the course content (Enos & Troppe, 1996). The Health Professions Schools In Service to the Nation (HPSISN) project provided support for this approach. In the evaluation summary of the first 2 years of its national service-learning project, HPSISN reported that course-based service-learning had the greatest transformational impact on students (HPSISN, 1997). During the visit, the evaluators added that "Students were strongly affected by working with individuals in non-clinical settings where they could learn about the daily context of individuals' lives, and experience the complex and fragile network of support services on which they depend" (p. 4). In structuring the service-learning experience, faculty should strive to select sites that best meet the course objectives. These will differ according to the level of the course. Having a variety of choices is important for freshmen, who are curious about all aspects of the nursing profession. For seniors, a more focused community experience that allowed them the opportunity to make a contribution to the community was more appropriate. Matching service experiences with course objectives gave students the greatest opportunities to succeed.

Through service-learning experiences, students gain awareness of a variety of circumstances that have impact on the health and well-being of those they serve. Nursing students in the clinical setting frequently encounter individuals (patients) in "artificial settings," dressed alike, attached to equipment that restricts their mobility, and experiencing a myriad of discomforts that limit their ability to express their true selves. In nonclinical settings, students can focus on a holistic assessment and be free from concerns about learning and applying clinical skills (HPSISN,

1997). For example, in the hospital, students care for patients who are living with HIV. In the service-learning experience, students serve along with outreach workers going door-to-door distributing HIV prevention information, and learning about the living environment of vulnerable groups who may be at risk for HIV infection. In their journals and reaction papers, students are asked to describe how the service experience influenced their academic lives. Comments include:

> I could relate what I learned in child psychology classes to my work at the day care center. I learned that I want to work with children.
>
> Volunteering for hospice showed me that dying is a normal part of life. . . . I now realize that nursing is what I want to do with the rest of my life.
>
> In the nursing home, I saw how the professional nurse handles difficult situations. I learned . . . the importance of a smile. I had made a positive difference in someone's life . . . and nothing is more important than that.
>
> Working with teenage mothers helped me learn how to relate to people from different backgrounds than my own. Service activities force you to go into the community and get to know what is around you.
>
> I have overcome my fears about working with disabled people . . . enabling me to grow within myself. We learn about real life outside of the classroom.

Clearly, student comments reflect the valuable aspects of the service-learning experience, especially when connected to academic learning.

CONNECTING ACADEMICS WITH COMMUNITY SERVICE

The overall program objectives of a nursing curriculum are the foundation for course objectives and learning activities. Objectives for individual courses are derived from the broad program objectives. Courses that incorporate service-learning have specific objectives related to the service requirement. The nursing faculty believed that through service-learning, students could meet more than simply the service-learning objective in each course. To validate this assumption, we surveyed students to see if they could connect their service experiences with the program objectives. Their responses to a written survey confirmed our impressions. Students in each level of the program reported that their service experiences had, indeed, helped them to meet the program objectives. Table 2.1 summarizes their responses. Students who returned the survey had service experiences in a variety of settings, yet were able to relate their learning to similar objectives. For instance, activities at the Boys and Girls Club, Hospice, and the Teenage Mothers Program helped students develop a personal philosophy for nursing practice. The majority of students responding to the survey identified opportunities that helped them to develop their communication skills. These opportunities included active listening; open-ended questioning; and therapeutic silence. Serving the community helped students to learn to appreciate differences and respect the dignity of those served. Students learned to appreciate the multiple roles of the nurse as collaborator, advocate, and researcher. They were introduced to holistic nursing practice in varied settings, from health promotion as peer educators to end-of-life care as hospice volunteers. Students were able to develop clinical skills through observation and hands-on care as part of the nursing team. Seniors recognized the importance of applying the nursing process in providing education to teenage mothers.

As nurse educators, we are faced with the challenge of preparing future generations of nurses who must be flexible and willing to serve the needs of a rapidly changing society. Service-learning is a way to meet that goal. By requiring community service, faculty start the process. By connecting the service to learning, a meaningful component of the professional nurse's role is cultivated. This cultivation is accomplished through guided reflection, dialogue journals, reaction papers, and student presentations. Examples of these techniques are presented in Chapter Three. Our evaluation of the work thus far is most promising.

Implementing the Program

Successful service-learning programs are based on comprehensive and thoughtful planning. Bringle and Hatcher (1996) outlined a comprehensive plan for implementing a program. They described a model for program implementation, The Comprehensive Action Plan for Service Learning (CAPSL), that was the result of the experiences of 44 institutions involved in the Campus Compact Project. This 10-step plan was similar to the plan followed by our nursing faculty at the University of Scranton. What was implemented by our faculty and how it worked are presented in the following pages. The University of Scranton, Department of Nursing

Table 2.1. Service-learning: Relationship to Program Objectives

Program Objective	Sophomores	Juniors	Seniors
Integrate a personal philosophy for nursing practice based on the uniqueness, worth, and dignity of human beings	Gave the students an appreciation of people from different backgrounds than their own. They could recognize individual uniqueness.	Helped students to develop a personal philosophy of caring. In the hospice setting, students developed respect for the dignity of their patients.	Were able to increase the self-esteem of those that they taught in peer education and the Teenage Mothers program.
Assume responsibility and accountability for evaluating one's own practice in relationship to accepted standards of nursing practice	Learned the importance of communication skills.	The hospice nurses served as excellent examples of professional nursing. Students learned the importance of a safe environment for patients.	Were able to identify standards for health promotion activities.
Synthesize theoretical principles applicable to professional nursing practice	Had an opportunity to relate to patients in a professional manner and engage in health teaching.	Observed the role of the nurse in patient teaching, pain management, and skill performance.	Learning the importance of the self-care model.
Utilize the nursing process to promote, restore, and maintain adaptation in individuals, families, communities and groups throughout the life cycle	Recognized the importance of health promotion through education with school -age girls and boys.	Promoted adaptation through hospice care.	Applied the nursing process to provide education to teenage mothers.
Collaborate with clients, colleagues, and the public to assure optimal health and welfare of clients	Reported to the nursing manager at the service agency.	Collaborated with nurses in hospice care and with patients. Advocated for children at the community club.	Increase their skills for effective collaboration in planning peer education programs.
Assume responsibility and accountability in providing comprehensive health care	Learned responsibility in the care of children in day care.	Gave comprehensive care to patients in the hospice setting.	Used a holistic focus in peer education.

continued

Table 2.1. *(continued)*

Program Objective	Sophomores	Juniors	Seniors
Evaluate interpersonal skills when communicating with individuals, families, communities and groups	Improved their communication skills. Learned to be active listeners. Connected with the experiences of young children in today's world.	Used open-ended questioning effectively. Learned the benefit of therapeutic silence in hospice. Improved communication skills with the elderly. Overcame phobia of public speaking.	Improved skills in communicating with a variety of community groups.
Incorporate pertinent research findings in refining and extending one's own nursing practice	Learned to be open to the ideas of others.	No opportunity	Were able to recognize areas in need of research.
Continue personal and professional growth	Gained insight into themselves, and why they chose nursing. Continued to participate in service even though the required hours were completed.	Through the observation of nurses they were able to improve their own skills which helped to secure a summer internship. Gave them an opportunity to give back to the community.	Teaching in the peer education program helped to develop professionally.

was extremely fortunate to be selected as one of twenty schools nationally to receive funding from the Pew Charitable Trusts "Health Professions Schools In Service to the Nation" program. The 3-year grant provided the funding needed to launch a successful service-learning program.

The first step was to establish a planning group. Ideally it should be composed of representatives from faculty, administration, staff, students, and community partners who will develop the strategy for implementation. The individuals selected should be enthusiastic about service-learning and capable of inspiring others to join the program and promote service-learning. The program should reflect the mission of the institution, the college, and the academic department. Service-learning is a natural match for many universities, since most are committed to service to the community as part of their mission. If not, it is important that a service commitment be established that will support service-learning in the institution. The mission and goals of the University of Scranton stress its dedication to serving others. The J. A. Panuska College of Professional Studies requires community service for all students, and the philosophy of the department of nursing encourages students to be involved in community service. With this as our foundation, service-learning fit naturally into our curriculum. In addition to nursing faculty and students, the planning group included the Dean of the J. A. Panuska College of Professional Studies, the director of Collegiate Volunteers, and several community agency representatives.

The second step focused on increasing campus and community awareness of the goals of service-learning. This can be accomplished in several ways: 1) support faculty to attend service-learning conferences; 2) provide service-learning seminars on campus; 3) join national service-learning organizations; and 4) invite community partners to seminars and conferences. Both the HPSISN grant and the University of Scranton administration provided funds for several faculty, each year, to participate in regional and national conferences. During the second year of the program, an internal grant supported a one-day seminar presented by a national expert on service-learning for all members of the university community. Jacoby (1996) reported over 50 national organizations that support service-learning. The J. A. Panuska College of Professional Studies at the University of Scranton is a member of the Community-Campus Partnerships for Health (CCPH), an organization formed in 1996 for health professions schools interested in community-based education. The National League for Nursing also is committed to community-based nursing education.

The third step suggests that consultations with outstanding programs be planned. Service-learning was initiated in the 1960s, and many excellent programs are in existence today. The literature is replete with numerous examples from a variety of disciplines. Being one of 20 grantee schools in the HPSISN program provided ample opportunities to network and consult with both experts and novices to plan our strategy. (See Appendix A for a list of resources).

Resource allocation is the fourth step in program planning. Certainly, administrative support is critical in this area, and includes funding for a service-learning director, an office of service-learning, and staff to administer, monitor, and evaluate the program. Several authors describe alternate sources of funding, with grant money being most often cited (Leder & McGuinness, 1996; Morton, 1996). Funding can be directed to faculty and staff salaries and development activities, stipends for graduate assistants to help monitor the program, and equipment for offices and service-learning materials. In addition to national sources for funding, private foundations and individual donors can be valuable sources of support. Providing adequate resources for service-learning sends an important message to faculty that their work is valued, thereby encouraging other faculty to partake in service-learning.

Bringle and Hatcher (1996) list expansion as the fifth step for a successful program. Faculty development, and the funding of conferences, and on-campus seminars about service-learning, serves to spread the word that service-learning is a meaningful addition to the curriculum. As previously mentioned, at the University of Scranton, the nursing department hosted a campus-wide service-learning seminar featuring Dr. Richard Couto, funded through an internal grant. The sixth step is recognition, which is easily accomplished through media including service-learning newsletters; local newspaper coverage of service activities; and scholarly publications.

Program monitoring and evaluation are no strangers to nursing faculty, and are an expected part of the plan. Service-learning outcomes should be part of each course evaluation. Overall service-learning statistics tallying the number of students participating, the number of agencies served, and the number of service hours provided are all important data. At the University of Scranton over the past 3 years, the number of service hours increased from 1,570 hours in 1996 to almost 3,000 hours in 1998. The annual program evaluation is shared with the University administration and is included in the Department's annual report. During the academic year, regular service-learning reports are given to faculty at department meetings. The evaluation tools are included in Appendices B, C, and D. Feedback on evaluation should be shared with the community agencies. This subject is discussed in greater detail in Chapter Five.

Evaluation data is crucial and provides the foundation for program growth. Research is the natural next step in the process. There are opportunities to share at regional and national conferences. Involving students in the research plan is an added benefit. During the past 3 years, University of Scranton students have presented at national conferences on topics including: service-learning program evaluation; HIV education outcomes for high school and college students; and HIV Women's Outreach (see below). As faculty connect their research and service interests, opportunities for mentoring and scholarship will flourish (Giles & Eyler, 1994; Leder & McGuinness, 1996; Zlotkowski, 1996).

The final step in planning a service-learning curriculum is institution-alization. According to Bringle and Hatcher (1996), developing the program from the institution's mission is crucial for success. Service-learning courses can start in general education courses, or, as in our case, be initiated by an individual department or division of the university. Either way, results must be shared across the campus, the community, and with other universities. The benefits are contagious, and the best vehicles for dissemination are the students, whose enthusiasm and commitment are, truly, the winds beneath our wings.

Another strategy is identifying community agencies, i.e., surveying community agencies for applicable projects for the students. Rather than creating new projects, join existing ones. Community agencies are often short-staffed and, with the help of a university partnership, they are able to offer programs that otherwise might not be possible. One example was an HIV Women's Outreach program in Northeastern Pennsylvania coordinated by the American Red Cross. Students in the senior-level community health nursing course chose this work as their service project for the fall semester. They were so successful that they returned in the spring semester (when the service was no longer a course requirement) and moved the project from community information sessions to direct door-to-door outreach efforts with vulnerable women. Working in teams with nursing faculty and Red Cross outreach workers, the students were able to offer HIV prevention information to over 400 women in a 4-week period. Without the students' involvement, the Red Cross outreach coordinator would not have been able to reach more than 100 women in the same time period.

FACULTY RESPONSIBILITY

When all is said and done, faculty are central to the implementation of service-learning. As previously discussed, without faculty interest, service-learning cannot be developed (Bringle & Hatcher, 1996; Stanton, 1991; Wills, 1992). Students can serve the community through cocurricular sponsors, but the connection to learning will be lost. Faculty are key to course integration and successful student outcomes. Faculty responsibilities are numerous and include: reading and returning journals (with feedback); connecting with community agency staff to coordinate orientation and evaluation of students; and monitoring completion of service hours. In addition to regular course assignments, students will be writing dialogue journals and reaction papers about their service activities. Returning the journal on a regular basis gives the student important feedback and potentiates learning. Support from the campus service coordinator, graduate assistants, and student leaders is most helpful.

Benefits to Faculty

Incorporating service-learning brings added faculty responsibilities, but it also can hold many rewards. At the University of Scranton it gave us increased visibility in the community. The local newspaper highlighted articles on hospice and middle and high school HIV-prevention education projects in which our students were involved. The media focus stimulated faculty interest and breathed new life into existing faculty-sponsored service activities. The service-learning program advertised existing programs to students, and offered assistance to faculty who were engaged in separate service activities. It stimulated faculty thinking about and eventual acceptance of the need for curriculum reform to a more community-based learning model. It created opportunities to partner not only with service agencies, but with our nursing colleagues at neighboring universities. The department received one grant for a joint project and submitted a proposal to work with five other institutions to plan community-based nursing education at a community site. Our success in service-learning provided a starting point for discussions with related disciplines in our college, such as physical therapy, occupational therapy, counseling, human services, and health administration.

SUMMARY

This chapter examined service-learning and its integration into the nursing curriculum, a challenging task that is certainly worth the effort. Models for implementation were presented and examples from experiences at the University of Scranton were highlighted. While administrative support and faculty commitment are crucial elements to the success of service-learning, the experiences of the students—introduced to the realities of life for the disadvantaged, the disabled, the most vulnerable of our society—are the foundation of our success. Students reflect on their experiences through writing journals and papers. Methods for successful utilization of reflection techniques are presented in Chapter Three.

REFERENCES

Bringle, R. G., & Hatcher, J. A. (1996). Implementing service learning in higher education. *Journal of Higher Education, 67*(2), 221–239.

Buchen, I. H. (1995). Service learning and curriculum transfusion. *NASSP Bulletin*, Volume 79 Issue #564, 66–70.

Clark, P. G., Spence, D. L., & Sheehan, J. L. (1987). A service/learning model for interdisciplinary teamwork in health and aging. *Gerontology & Geriatrics Education, 6*(4), 3–16.

Darbyshire, P. (1994). Understanding caring through arts and humanities: A medical/nursing humanities approach to promoting alternative experiences of thinking and learning. *Journal of Advanced Nursing, 19*, 856–863.

Enos, S. L., & Troppe, M. L. (1996). Service-learning in the curriculum. In B. Jacoby, & Associates (Eds). *Service-learning in higher education: Concepts and practices.* (pp.). San Francisco: Jossey-Bass.

Giles, D. E., & Eyler, J. (1994). The impact of a college community service laboratory on students' personal, social and cognitive outcomes. *Journal of Adolescence, 17*, 327–39.

Hales, A. (1997). Service-learning within the nursing curriculum. *Nurse Educator, 22*(2), 15–18.

HPSISN, (1997). *Health professions schools in service to the nation: 1996–1997 evaluation report.* Portland State University.

Jacoby, B. & Associates (1996). *Service-learning in higher education.* San Francisco: Jossey-Bass.

Leder, D., & McGuinness, I. (1996). Making the paradigm shift: Service learning in higher education. *Metropolitan Universities*, 47–56.

Morton, K. (1996). Issues related to integrating service-learning into the curriculum. In B. Jacoby Associates (Eds). *Service-learning in higher education: Concepts and practices* (pp. 276–296). San Francisco: Jossey-Bass.

Porter, J. R., & Schwartz, L. B. (1993). Experiential service-based learning: An integrated HIV/AIDS education model for college campuses. *Teaching Sociology, 21*, 409–415.

Stanton, T. K. (1991). Liberal arts, experiential learning and public service: Necessary ingredients for socially responsible undergraduate education. *Journal of Cooperative Education, 27*(2), 55–68.

Wills, J. R. (1992). Service: On campus and the curriculum. *Educational Record*, Volume 73 Issue #2, 32–36.

Zlotkowski, E. (1996). A new voice at the table? Linking service-learning and the academy. *Change*, Volume 28 Issue #1, 20–27.

CHAPTER 3

Critical Reflection

Patricia A. Bailey, Ed.D., R.N. C.S.

Experience alone will not educate the student—it must
be supported by the reflective thought process

—Anonymous

At this point in the text, it should be clear that a service-learning program
is unique in many ways, and is different than learning through our well-
developed clinical experiences. Critical reflection is one important aspect
of service-learning that is essential to the educational process. Faculty in
nursing will generally be comfortable with engaging in the reflective
process with students, since they do this in varied ways as they guide students through the clinical practice setting. However, there are many techniques available for faculty to use in approaching "critical reflection" that
will facilitate the learning process for students engaged in service. Chapter
Three stresses the process of connecting the student with learning through
the reflective process, describes various techniques for reflection, and discusses the link of reflection with critical thinking. Examples from journals
written by students serve as proof that students do indeed learn from their
service and are able to show this through the reflective process.

CONNECTING THROUGH REFLECTION

In his work on experiential learning, Kolb (1984) defines learning as "the process whereby knowledge is created through the transformation of experience" (p. 38). As students begin to become involved in service-learning experiences, it quickly becomes evident to them that they need to talk about and share what is happening in their community contacts. Although many will share their experiences with other students and friends and perhaps even family members in an informal way, a gap will exist between the service being given and the learning environment in the academic setting. Reflection experiences will help fill this gap and will assist the student and faculty member come to a better understanding of the learning that is taking place outside the class and how it is enhancing the formal academic experience. In discussing the importance of "reflective learning", Boyd and Fales (1983) defined reflection as

> the *process* of creating and clarifying the meaning of experience (present or past) in terms of self (self in relation to self and self in relation to the world). The outcome of the process is changed conceptual perspective. The experience that is explored and examined to create meaning focuses around or embodies a concern of central importance to the self (p. 101).

In his book, *The Call of Service*, Coles (1993) emphasizes the importance of reflection:

> Our institutions of higher learning might certainly take heed, not only by encouraging students to do such service, but by helping them stop and mull over, through books and discussions, what they have heard and seen. This is the purpose, after all, of colleges and universities-to help one generation after another grow intellectually and morally through study and the self-scrutiny such study can sometimes prompt (p. 148).

Reflection is not a new concept for those in academia. Part of everyone's clinical experience is getting the student to think about what they are doing and to critically analyze the connections between theory and practice, that is, how to connect what one does in practice to what is taught in the classroom and published in the texts. Saylor (1990) reminds us that

reflection provides the opportunity for appropriate self-evaluation necessary for high professional standards. In addition, systematic reflection
increases the possibility that one will draw accurate conclusions from
clinical experiences (p. 11).

Others see reflection as

separating elements in the experience (analysis) and connecting those
elements with other experiences and knowledge (synthesis), as well as
other mental activities, such as feeling emotions (Horwood, 1995, p. 27).

When students engage others in the community, they do so for various
reasons, not least of which is their desire to care for those in need of some
type of service. Faculty see this "caring" behavior often in the planned
clinical settings, and can help students define and identify their roles as
caring professionals in a formal clinical setting. However, as students
become involved in service-learning in various community sites, the faculty member is most often not there to see student behaviors, and therefore
the feedback on helping students interpret what is happening to them may
be absent. Students need help in interpreting what is going on in the community experience and need to be able to talk about it with the faculty,
community agency personnel, and their peers.

Reflection is a critical component of the service-learning process. It
enables the student to make the connections between service in the community and their learning experiences in the academic setting. It also gives
them the opportunity to examine their attitudes and value systems in relation to others . As we begin to engage students in the service experience,
it is important to remember that there needs to be a "preparation" and
"preservice reflection" time built into the orientation process. Students
need information about the agency they will be engaged in, the clients
being served by that agency or service, and the expected role performance
of students in that service experience. This information-sharing may take
place in the service setting and may be led by agency personnel. However,
it is important to spend some academic time in the classroom setting to
further explore with students their anxieties, concerns, myths, and other
issues that may surface. Students need help in building a bridge from the
service they are engaged in to the learning that is taking place in the more
formal setting—the college environment. Jacoby (1996) points to the
importance of reflection if the service-learning experience is to enhance

learning and address community needs, and stresses that "reflection and reciprocity are key concepts of service-learning" (p. 5). Planning for critical reflection sessions will provide the opportunity for students to explore what is happening in their service experiences and to make the connections necessary for enhanced lifelong learning.

TECHNIQUES FOR REFLECTION

There are many ways one can help students reflect, and faculty need to be creative in designing ways that best meet their skills and the needs of students. There are various definitions for the "reflective process" found in the literature. Some examples are:

> the process of reviewing one's repertoire of clinical experience and knowledge to invent novel approaches to complex clinical problems. Reflection also provides data for self examination and increases learning from experience.
>
> As part of the processing of raw experience, reflection engages students in consciously thinking about their experiences and provides an opportunity for them to examine and question values and beliefs and to develop problem solving skills (Silcox, 1995, p. 46).

Some popular methods for reflection include classroom discussion, student journal-writing, focus groups, audio/visual presentations, portfolios , shared readings on "community" topics, and end-of-semester reaction papers. This is not an exhaustive list, and faculty need to be encouraged to develop new, creative ways for students to reflect on service and how it directs their academic and personal lives. If the term "reflection" is not a comfortable one for students or for faculty, other terms can be used, such as "group discussion", "thoughts and ideas", or "time out". However, it is important that students know from the beginning that reflection in some form is essential to the process of learning from the service experience. Since not all students will feel comfortable sharing their experiences and feelings, by providing a variety of ways for reflection, every student will have the opportunity to reflect in a way that is most comfortable for them.

Classroom Discussion

Conducting reflection through classroom discussion is best accomplished with small groups of between 8–12 students. Arranging chairs in a circle is essential so that all participants can see each other and can freely talk and listen. If faculty are engaging in this for the first time, they may decide they want someone with more experience in group discussions to lead the reflection. Resource personnel may be found in any one of the following groups on campus: Student Affairs, Counseling Center, Campus Ministry, and graduate students from departments such as Psychology, Counseling, and Social Services. However, nursing faculty input and participation is essential if the student is to be helped to see the connections between service and the nursing curriculum. Encouraging student participation is also essential, and initially the facilitator of a group can start by asking everyone to mention what service activity they are engaged in. After this, students can be asked to describe in "one word" their overall reaction to the experience. Comments from students such as "wonderful", "scared", "exhausting", "fulfilling" will facilitate further dialogue and discussion among the group. Following are some possible questions to ask students to respond to, and some past responses from freshmen and sophomore nursing students who were engaged in a service-learning experience:

What expectations or myths did you have prior to the experience?
Scared of nursing homes, expected to work with the elderly at the soup kitchen but not children, thought the people would be sad and depressed, had many myths about HIV infection

Describe the most enjoyable aspect of your experience.
Helping people, I made a difference, watching nurses and doctors work as a team, communicating with patients and staff

Describe the most frustrating aspect of your experience.
Finding time for the service, the families did not visit the residents, there were not enough nurses, that the patient got upset remembering the past

Describe the most surprising aspect of your experience.
How nice the facility was, that I had prior prejudices, the friends I made, that I was highly regarded as a volunteer

What have you learned about yourself?
Had patience, did not want to be a nurse, can interact with strangers successfully, I'll make a good nurse

What have you learned about the needs of this community?
Nursing homes are needed, nurses burn out, health care is complex, a need for more volunteers

What have you learned about society?
People neglect their families in nursing homes, we do not value the elderly, health care workers are not appreciated, society is interdisciplinary

What did you like/dislike about the community agency?
Liked: The staff, other volunteers, being told I was appreciated, the variety
Disliked: How long it took to get in touch with the agency, nursing home residents sat in chairs with nothing to do, tedious procedures

Has this experience changed your ideas of, or approaches to, interacting with people?
Become more tolerant, open-minded, need to be more patient, more of a need for holistic care

Have you felt useful as a volunteer?
Over 80% answered yes to this question

Describe how this service-learning has influenced your academic life.
Helps me apply what I learn, helps me budget my time, learned communication skills, interpersonal skills were enhanced

How has service-learning affected your personal life?
It was an emotional experience, had to deal with different people and a different community, know myself and my values better, someday I'll need help, made me feel confident and responsible

As one can see, students can and do engage in meaningful reflection, and given a supportive environment will verbalize their expectations and experiences in a group reflection session. As one looks over the above responses, it is very evident that students are going through varied learning experiences. Reflection is a time for faculty and other students to support each other and validate and reaffirm what each is experiencing.

Marquette University has developed a reflection guide that can be useful for students to use in writing a journal or in group reflection sessions:

Orientation: Who am I? Why am I here? What is important to me? Where do I come from?

Observation: What do I see and hear? How do I describe what I see through storytelling and facing the problem)?

Feelings: How do I feel about what I see and hear? Why do I feel this way?

Interpretation: Why did I see what I saw? How do my values and experiences as part of a certain cultural, racial, ethnic, religious group, etc., shape what I see and hear? What are the barriers that prevent me from changing?

Personal Analysis: How am I part of the problem? How have I worked to be part of the solution? What gifts can I offer or learn? Where can I draw hope and strength? What signs of hope exist?

Social Analysis: What are the social and political roots of the problem? What are the possible solutions? Who holds power in this society? How can we as a group become empowered for change? What agency/institution holds the most hope for changing the current situation? (Jacoby, 1996, p. 141).

There is no magic number of times that classroom reflection should occur during the semester, however, a group reflection at mid-semester and another at the end of the semester seems appropriate. Discussion should last for the class period, but for no longer than 1 hour. Each faculty member needs to evaluate this for themselves. Based on specific program needs, faculty may decide to conduct a reflection session outside of class time. This can be arranged in the evenings, in conjunction with a nursing association meeting, or perhaps the session can take place in the community agency where a group of students are engaged. This is a great way to engage community partners in the reflection and strengthen campus-community relationships. This will be further discussed in Chapter Five. You may want to take some notes during this reflection discussion, but if so, it is best to have a recorder for just that purpose. One could also have the students jot down their thoughts to specific questions and collect these at the end of the discussion. Generally, these written responses would be anonymous, so students can feel free to share (See Appendix C for Forms for Reflection).

Student Journal Writing

Journal writing is an excellent method for having the students explore their own behavior and their interactions in the service experience. It is a way for them to make sense of what they are doing in a particular agency, and when the journal is read by faculty, it gives the faculty person the opportunity to intervene in situations that may be undesirable for students' learning. A common theme among those advocates of journal writing is: you don't learn from experience—you learn by reflecting on your experiences! Nurse educators have used the "journal" experience as a way to help students reflect "attitudes, feelings, and expansion of his or her cognitive learning throughout the nursing course" (Callister, 1993, p. 185). More recently in nursing education, there has been a stress on enhancing critical thinking skills among students, and the clinical journal has been utilized as one method to foster critical thinking skills. Brown and Sorrell (1993) point out;

> An important purpose of the clinical journal is to provide guided opportunities for students to "think aloud" on paper, reflecting on their own perceptions or understandings of the situations they encounter in the practicum (p. 16).

Journal writing for service-learning experiences has very similar objectives as when used in other circumstances. Before beginning the journal, it is helpful to have students examine their preconceptions and expectations before they start their service-learning experience. An effective way to do this is to have the students write a letter to themselves. They can be directed to answer certain questions such as:

> Before I start this experience I have the following expectations about this community agency. . . .
> I believe I can contribute the following to this community service. . . .
> I have the following concerns. . . .
> I think the needs of this agency are. . . .

The letter can be sealed and kept by the faculty member or by each student. At the end of the service experience and perhaps at the last group reflection, students can read their letters and reflect on what their pre-service ideas and concerns were. This can be shared, if the group is so inclined, or read privately and reflected on prior to completing a final reflection paper or other service assignment for the course.

A very effective type of journal writing for service experiences is the dialogue journal. Students write in their journal after each service contact. The journal is then shared with the course faculty, and the faculty person writes back to the student in the student's journal. Several criteria need to be considered if this type of reflection is to prove beneficial. The student and faculty member must be conscientious in submitting the journal on time. The purpose of writing after each contact is to give the student the opportunity to reflect immediately after the experience and not lose significant pieces of the service experience. In turn, the faculty person reading the journal needs to respond quickly to the student's reflection in order to maintain meaningful feedback. This is a time-consuming exercise, but one that has proven to be extremely beneficial to both student reflection and faculty input into the learning process.

In some instances, it may be possible to have someone beside the course faculty read the journals and reflect back to the student. For example, a course graduate assistant or another faculty person may be given reassigned time to read student journals. If this is done, there needs to be ongoing interaction between the person reading the journals and the course faculty member in order to assure the connections between service in the community and learning based on course objectives. In other words, the student needs to see the connection between what they are doing in their service experiences and how this is contributing to their academic learning. On some campuses there may be a student volunteer center. If this is the case, a faculty member wishing to include a service-learning experience may be able to negotiate with the volunteer center to assist with reflections in class and also to help with reading the dialogue journals. If this is done, it is essential that the same person read the same student's journal for the entire semester. This will support the development of a relationship between student and reader that is beneficial to all.

If the faculty member reading the journal is not the faculty person teaching the course, the student must be informed of this at the very beginning of the semester. If students have concerns about whom is reading their journal, the faculty person is responsible for doing all that is possible to accommodate the student.

Other situations can be established for journal writing. A group journal can be initiated if a number of students are writing on one particular service experience. The journal can be kept at a library reference desk or in some other secure environment. Students write in the journal at specific times and everyone can read each other's journal entry. This becomes a "dialogue" among the students. The faculty member can also participate.

On some campuses, there are "theme" houses. If there was a community service or volunteer house, students living in that house could develop a journal writing club. This could involve students pairing off and sharing their journal with each other throughout the course of a service-learning experience. Later on in this chapter, methods for writing journals will be addressed.

Freshmen students in their first nursing course and service-learning experience expressed concerns in their journals regarding visiting the elderly in long-term care facilities and in general hospitals. They felt they would be "uncomfortable trying to talk with them" and thought the clients themselves "would not accept them". As the experience ended, students reflected on what actually happened: they felt needed, the residents looked forward to their visit, and the students looked forward to being with the resident and sharing their student life experiences with them . Students felt they actually had "something to offer" to the elderly. Students were able to share their vision of the professional nursing role as they were interacting in the community, and were able to compare it to discussions in the classroom regarding professional role content.

Senior students in their Community Health course had their community assessment project combined with a service-learning experience which involved assessment of the needs and resources of elderly residents in a senior housing unit. Journal entries included: "We are able to thoroughly assess the resources provided to the residents and we have identified an area of 'social activity' as a need for this age group". Another student serving in a soup kitchen for the homeless wrote, "I am better able to relate to people because of this experience;" "I am becoming more accustomed to different cultures;" and "It has helped me think differently about family values". Some students who worked in a Teenage Mothers Program in a local school system reflected, "I am just trying to get them to trust me;" and "Writing this journal does make me realize that sometimes we do make a difference, even if it is to just one teenage mom."

In reading student journals, it is evident that although some students may experience difficult situations in a service-learning setting, all students generally are able to reflect on changes in themselves, and are able to experience an increased understanding of the needs of those they come in contact with in the community. This is clearly pointed out by Goldsmith (1995):

> When service participants take the time to examine their service experiences closely, they gain a deeper and more thorough understanding and accounting of events than when they simply perform the tasks without reflection. Reflection offers an opportunity to step back and review both

individual and group accomplishments and progress. In their journals, participants can recognize and acknowledge their own strengths, and identify and explore weaknesses. Journal reflection also offers an opportunity to assess and celebrate one's impact on others (p. 4–5).

The following journal entry from a freshman nursing student demonstrates the learning and growth that occurs:

> This semester I chose to spend my service-learning hours at the Veteran's Center. I was a bit nervous on my first day, even though my job was as easy as a game of bingo. I was a little hesitant at first with the idea of working with the elderly. I was afraid that it would be difficult to communicate with them and they might even give me a hard time. Today, however, my goal was to conquer this fear.
>
> My first task was to help bring the residents to the multi-purpose room for a game of bingo. As soon as I pushed my first wheelchair and had a conversation with John, I knew everything would be all right. We talked about how beautiful the weather was and he explained to me that he had started a "fund" for his new granddaughter with his 50-cent bingo winnings. During the game, I sat with a man that couldn't move his arms too well, so we played together and won several times! I met many of the other volunteers who seem to really care. Many of them know the residents on a first-name basis. I hope to get more involved with the nursing staff in the future.
>
> My first day was a wonderful experience. I immediately realized that many of the thoughts we have about the elderly are really misconceptions. I can't wait to go back!

Focus Groups

Selected group discussion is another technique used to facilitate reflection around a specific topic. Simply stated, it involves small groups of individuals, 6 to 12 people, coming together for a specific time period of about 1 to 2 hours to focus on a specific topic through a common dialogue and exchange of ideas. More commonly seen as a method for collecting data for a qualitative research study, "focus groups are basically group interviews . . . the reliance is on interaction within the group, based on topics that are supplied by the researcher who typically takes the role of a moderator"(Morgan, 1997, p. 2). Although you may not be considering collecting data for research, by focusing members of a group on specific elements of a service-learning experience, a more varied interpretation of the experience may emerge. All members of the group will benefit from this form of sharing. There is generally a facilitator for the group and some guidelines to focus the discussion and allow for a summary or conclusions to come from the group. Focus groups have been successful as a method of getting a "mixed" group to reflect on a service-learning experience. For example, having community partners, faculty, and students come together to focus on what is happening in a particular community agency, or to critically think together and reflect on how service-learning is impacting on the community and the learning of students. Stevens (1996) discusses focus groups and understanding community health issues and stresses, "A main advantage of focus-group interviewing is the possibility of stimulating spontaneous exchanges of ideas, experiences, and attitudes in an atmosphere that can be safer . . . given the solidarity of the group" (p. 171). This is an excellent way to foster community relationships and to engage all "players" in a service-learning project to critically reflect on the outcomes of the service experience. For more information on using focus groups in service-learning programs, the reader is referred to the works of Richard A. Krueger (1988) and David L. Morgan (1997).

Audio/Visual Presentations

Multimedia techniques offer varied ways for students to reflect on their service experiences. Having students develop a photo, video, or slide presentation in conjunction with their service-learning supports a creative way for students to engage in the reflective process. By presenting to other groups of students, faculty, or agency personnel, further discussion and dialogue on the service experience is facilitated . Often, new ideas and insights will emerge from this in-depth creative process. A less time-consuming reflective process could include painting, drawing, or developing an individual collage of one's service experience. This could take place in or outside of class, requires a relatively short span of time, and is easily shared during a reflection session with other students, faculty, or agency partners. Students can be asked to draw symbolically what the service experience has meant to them and then to describe this to the group. Another example of using creative talents to reflect on service is to have students create a dance, a piece of music, or a theater presentation to visualize their experience of service. There may be students in nursing who are talented in the arts, and who would welcome the opportunity to express themselves in a more creative environment. Writing for a service-learning newsletter, a college newspaper, or preparation of a student-written manuscript for publication are others ways in which reflection can occur. Students can also be encouraged to develop poster presentations of their work in service to the community. Posters can be displayed locally in the academic and community setting or be submitted for presentations at regional and national conferences. All of the above require faculty support and facilitation for meaningful reflection to occur.

Portfolios

Designing a portfolio can be very time-consuming for students, but at the same time, it offers them the opportunity to reflect over time on their experiences while engaged in service-learning. Gordon (1994) describes portfolios as "a compendium of work in any format (visual, verbal, written, musical, symbolic, and the like) which reflect student learning and growth during the semester" (p. 23). Criteria for what should be included in the portfolio need to be established at the beginning of the service-learning experience. This may include journal writing, service objectives, connections to course content, artistic presentations, or symbolic interpretations of the service experience. It is helpful for students to have some discussion regarding the development of their portfolios as the semester progresses. Because of the work involved for each student, a reasonable portion of the course grade should be allocated for the portfolio. Students can present their portfolios to the class and the evaluation process can include student critique and comment. This is an excellent way to have students reflect together on what an individual has learned from the service experience and a positive way to share ideas and insights to learning. Gordon and Julius (1995) stress the value of this reflective method;

> Portfolios touch the heart of education—inspiring students to demonstrate their growth while contributing to their continued learning. Rather than causing a break with other educational experiences, portfolios have become central to the learning process for our students, serving as a powerful tool to engage people of diverse ages, as we relate in this discussion of our work in two very different settings. (p. 94)

Shared Readings

Engaging students in reading a piece of literature is another way to help students reflect on what they are learning as they become involved in the service setting. Readings that relate to various aspects of a service experience can be assigned, and students can discuss their reactions to those readings, either in a group discussion, a focus group, a journal entry, or through a written reaction paper assignment. Kirkpatrick (1994) and Darbyshire (1995) share their experiences of using arts, literature, and newspapers in the teaching of nursing students. Faculty can be creative in choosing a particular reading by looking at fictional and nonfictional literature that will relate to service experiences students are involved in. For example, if students are engaged in serving an elderly population, they may be asked to read such works as *When I am an Old Woman I Shall Wear Purple* by Jenny Joseph (1994). If engaged in service with minorities, students can read any one of the following works: *Black Ice* by Lorene Cary (1991); *To Be Young, Gifted and Black* by Lorraine Hansberry and adapted by Robert Nemiroff (1969); *Days of Obligation: An Argument with My Mexican Father* by Richard Rodriguez (1992); *When I Was Puerto Rican* by Esmeralda Santiago (1993); or *Lame Deer: Seeker of Visions* by John (Fire) Lame Deer and Richard Erdoes (1972). These are just a few of the many literary pieces that could be read by students and then discussed further in a shared reading session. Valiga and Bruderle (1997) present in greater detail the use of the arts and humanities in the teaching of nursing;

> By integrating the arts and humanities into the teaching and learning experiences they design, faculty can enhance students' appreciation of the intensity of life, the diversity of their fellow human beings, and the richness of the world around them (p. 16).

Reaction Papers

Requiring short summary papers submitted at the end of the semester is an excellent way to have the student reflect back over the semester and pull together what has been learned and valued from the service experience. A 3–4 page paper is appropriate for this assignment. Students can be asked to include the following:

- Describe the experience. Where? What did you do?
- What did you learn about yourself?
- What did you learn about the community?
- What was the most enjoyable part?
- What was the least enjoyable part?
- Describe how learning in the community has had an impact on your academic life.

Following is an example of a reaction paper from a freshman nursing student who had chosen the Jewish Home of Eastern Pennsylvania for her service-learning *experience*:

> My duties as a volunteer were to feed the residents and provide them with company during my visits. I went to the Nursing Home every Saturday and volunteered a total of 151/2 hours.
>
> When I first started this project I was somewhat apprehensive of how well I would interact with the elderly. I remember thinking to myself, "What could I possibly give to an 85-year-old?" As the weeks passed by, this apprehension quickly disappeared. I began to feel at ease with the residents and actually enjoyed them. I began to realize that the elderly are people too, with the same fears and worries as the rest of society. After this revelation, I no longer looked at my volunteer hours as a chore, but as a learning experience where I learned not only about the residents but about myself as well.
>
> From service-learning I have realized that I am able to share myself with others and in the process deeply enjoy it! This project made me even more confident that I will be able to succeed as a nurse by being compassionate and nurturing. Not only have I benefited from this experience, but the community has too. By giving just a couple of hours a week, I have made many lives a bit brighter. Knowing that I have done this makes all the early morning visits worthwhile.
>
> The most enjoyable aspect of my time at the nursing home was the residents. Once they felt comfortable around me, they began to open up and share a part of themselves with me. I learned about their children, their culture, and their past. They came to depend on my presence, and when my requirement was up, I frequently wanted to stay with them longer, even if it was just to sit there and not say a word.
>
> Despite all the positive aspects that came out of this project, I also saw some things that saddened me. After all the Saturdays I spent there,

only once did I see a child of a resident come to visit. This daughter barely stayed 20 minutes. The daughter was unable to finish feeding her own mother and even looked uneasy being with her. This observation angered me, because our parents sacrifice so much for us and raise us our entire lives without even asking for repayment. I think the least we can do is love them and take care of them when they begin to age. The majority of the residents at the home I don't believe medically even belong there. The truth of the matter is that people today just do not have the time or do not want to make the time to take care of someone else. Learning in the community has impacted my life greatly at the University. To be able to take what I learn in the classroom and apply it to my service-learning has been an extremely rewarding experience. The classroom provides the information and the community enabled me to put this knowledge to work. Service-learning has helped me put my "feet in the water" and begin to see what the nursing profession is truly like. Volunteering has been instrumental in learning more about myself, my future profession, and the world around me. All these aspects could never be learned in the classroom alone. (Faith A. Wobbe, Freshman Nursing Student, 1997)

WRITING A JOURNAL

Faculty need to explore the literature on "journal writing" to become familiar with the various types of journals that may be composed by students and to determine what standards are to be set to guide students in their writing. If faculty have never engaged in writing a journal, they need to set aside some time to focus on this activity for themselves. A weekly entry on what is happening with their teaching may be a good start. Another suggestion would be to journal about their clinical experience with clients in their practice setting. Perhaps a journal focus could be on their own service to the community and what ideas and insights come from that. Faculty need to experience "journal writing" before they attempt to journey with students along this path.

In *Journal Reflection: A Resource Guide for Community Service Leaders and Educators Engaged in Service Learning* (Goldsmith, 1995), various journal formats and approaches are described.

The personal journal is probably the most common one used. The student keeps his or her own book, and generally there are no set guidelines.

Anything can be written, and it is not shared with others. The advantage to this type of journal is that writers can be totally free with their expressions of reflections on the service experience. One does not have to be concerned that someone is going to read this and "What will they think of me?" Students who do not write well are not at a disadvantage, and can feel comfortable in the journaling process. Of course, there are some negative aspects of having students write personal journals. Since they are not shared, there is no feedback from others. Faculty will not know if students are writing in their journals or if they are even benefiting from this form of reflection. Some students do not feel they are learning or are on "the right track" if their journal is not shared and feedback is not given. Other benefits of journal writing, such as improved communication skills and critical thinking abilities, are not able to be assessed and encouraged.

The dialogue journal is a popular format for engaging students in the journal-writing process. In essence, the student writes in the journal and it is read by the faculty member (or some designee) and a written response on the journal entry is given back to the student. Both faculty and student engage in a dialogue about the student's service-learning experience. The journal is shared back and forth and a conversation is taking place between the two parties.

> The purpose of the dialogue journal is to create an environment in which two individuals can partake in an equal exchange. They can "talk" about anything—complaints, questions, thoughts, ideas, or interests, for example. For many people writing is more fun when they are assured that someone else will read and respond to what they have written. "Self expression", then, is no longer an abstract concept (Goldsmith, 1995, p. 23).

It is very important when engaged in a dialogue journal experience with students that both the journal writer and the reader have time to read, think about, and consider in detail what is happening in the service experience. This time element is essential for more meaningful responses and fruitful feedback from faculty to student. One of the most important elements when doing dialogue journals with students is to remember that what one reads is confidential and should be kept in confidence. It is a privilege that students allow us to read their journals, and initial orientation to the dialogue journal process should include information about confidentiality and respect for each of the two partners in this journaling. If students have difficulty with this concept, it may be best to chose another type of journal writing for the group.

Some general guidelines for responding to students in their journals are:

- Respond as soon as you receive the journal and return it to the student within a 3-day period. Attention to a quick turnaround time will foster interest and motivation on the part of students.
- Be generous in your comments, and avoid repetitious responses such as "That's good", or "Very interesting".
- Ask questions of your students. Keep in mind that the purpose of journal writing is to reflect, and that by questioning you will encourage further insights and ideas.
- Do not focus on correcting spelling and grammar mistakes. This is not the purpose of journal writing, and may discourage a student from writing freely about their insights and ideas.
- Be honest about what you think, but avoid pressing your views and opinions on the student. Encourage them to be open and honest about their thoughts and opinions of service.

Team journals can be used to engage a group of students who are involved in the same learning experience to share their journal writing. They will use the same book and can take turns writing an entry during the course of the semester. All members of the group have to have access to the journal and each student should read all entries. With this type of journal writing, members of the group respond to each other in addition to including their own reactions and insights to the service experience. A faculty member may join the group or not. Community-building and leadership skills can be strengthened through this type of activity.

Once you decide what type of journal to use with your students, criteria should be set so students have some guidance as to what should go into their journals. If you want to give them complete freedom in their writing, then you may only want to specify the number of journal entries you expect over a service learning experience. If you want them to address certain aspects of their experience, then you need to be specific with the criteria. The following is an example of criteria for a service-learning dialogue Journal for baccalaureate nursing students :

As part of your service-learning activities you will keep an ongoing journal account of your experience in a specific community service. Your journal entries should include the following for each contact:

1. Date and time spent in the community that day.
2. A description of your pre-experience attitudes regarding the specific community service you are engaged in.
3. An objective or goal for your contact that day.
4. Your personal reaction to the experience.
5. Comments about insights, new ideas, issues, points of confusion, etc.
6. Your thoughts and feelings regarding the experience.
7. Interactive experiences with other healthcare providers.
8. A description of your post-experience attitudes regarding the specific community service.
9. Comments regarding the experience and your role as a student in the nursing program. How is the experience relating to your academic studies?
10. Summarize, analyze, and evaluate your experience for the day.

Each faculty member has to decide what the journal writing goals and objectives are for their course. Criteria for writing the journal will flow from this.

REFLECTION AND CRITICAL THINKING

In nursing education, we have seen a gradual but consistent emphasis on the need to develop critical thinking skills in our upcoming practitioners. Both the National League for Nursing Accrediting Commission (1996) and the American Association of Colleges of Nursing (1998) have addressed the need for providing our students with learning experiences that will foster critical thinking skills. In the NLN criteria for the evaluation of baccalaureate programs (NLN, 1996) the required outcome criterion #1, Critical Thinking, states, "This outcome reflects students' skills in reasoning, analysis, research, and decision making relevant to the discipline of nursing"(p. 24). Others have stressed the connections between reflection and the critical thinking process and how learning is enhanced when one reflects and critically examines their interactions in a "real-world" experience (Mezirow, 1991; Mezirow & Associates, 1990; Schon, 1983; Sedlak, 1997).

Brown and Sorrell (1993) , Hahnemann (1986), and Callister (1993) point to the use of journal writing as a way of promoting critical thinking among our students. Given standard criteria for writing, students can be assisted through the critical thinking process of analysis of their service experience: "Students should be encouraged to document, summarize, analyze, and evaluate critical incidents..." (Brown & Sorrell, 1993, p. 18). It is through this reflective process in a service experience that students can engage in skills that reflect their ability to think critically:

> Broadly conceived, CT (critical thinking) can be characterized as purposeful, self-regulatory judgment, a human cognitive process. As such, CT is a pervasive human phenomenon that may be evident (at least on occasion) in problem solving, decision making, reasoned inquiry, professional practice, and everyday life (Facione & Facione, 1996, pp. 130–131).

Reflecting on one's service experience is a cognitive process. Students engaged in this process will reap the benefit of enhanced critical thinking skills and an expanded learning environment beyond the classroom setting. By reasoning about problems they encounter in the service experience and sharing this through thoughtful reflection, students and faculty will engage in that process of "shared learning" and thus will advance in the skill of critical thinking and reflection. Wong, Kember, Chung, and Yan (1995) studied the level of student reflection within their journal writing:

> We believe that we have established that the writing in reflective journals can be used to diagnose whether students are reflecting on their practice, and whether this reflection is critical in nature. Numerous courses in nursing education, as well as many fields of professional education, are now oriented towards promoting reflective thinking. A large proportion of these courses use reflective journals to encourage reflective thinking. The ability to analyze scripts for evidence of reflective thinking is, therefore, important. Unless it can be done in a reliable way it is difficult to establish whether the courses are achieving their aims and encouraging reflective thinking. (p. 56)

STUDENT VOICES

One of the easiest ways of evaluating the effectiveness of a service-learning experience is to listen to the voices of students! We end this chapter with some journal excerpts from nursing majors in a service-learning experience:

> I had a lot of fun and I can't wait to go back, but I will have to load up on coffee because those kids tired me out. It was really great because I talked to a Hispanic girl in Spanish. She helped me brush up for the Spanish test I had today.

> I suppose it is normal to have misconceptions about something you have never experienced. I was surprised about how many misconceptions I had about hospice. I was surprised at how "alive" someone who is dying can be! My personal life was affected by service-learning as well. The hospice experience showed me that I could be a support system for a sick patient without getting upset. Overall, the experience confirmed my desire to help others through the nursing profession.

> A goal I had set for myself today was to gain a better knowledge of the Jewish religion while watching this ceremony. I think that watching this ceremony was a very good experience for me. It helped me to recognize diversity in religion. This related to what I have learned in nursing class about cultural diversity and the different religions people have. I think it is important to accept everyone's religion since it plays a major role in many people's lives.

> Many residents don't realize how helpful and insightful they are to us students. When I mention it to them they are so surprised and I think it gives them a sense of self worth. These elderly women are definitely having an impact on my nursing knowledge. There is only so much you can learn from a book.

> Service-learning is a good thing for everyone to do at least once in their lifetime. It opens your eyes to a more wider perspective than our usual narrow view of "how we see things." Being a future health care provider it felt good to help in some small way, the community in which I live. After all, health care is about the whole person, not just the disease or people as statistics.

> This service-learning project enriched my academic life at the University. There are many times at college when I feel like I am isolated and my life does not extend beyond the campus. Activities like this force you to go into the community and get to know what is around you. The benefits are numerous.

SUMMARY

The reflective thought process stands out as the means whereby students can pull together what they learn in the service experience and its relationship to theoretical content. Faculty can help them make the connections between the service engaged in and curriculum content through journaling activities, reflective sessions, and focus groups. This chapter has focused on the meaning of reflection as an academic tool for student growth, both academically and personally. Various methods for reflection have been discussed and suggestions for guiding students in their journal writing have been explored. Students speak for themselves and share what they have learned and these are reflected in their journal entries. In Chapter Four, the promises and problems of service-learning are discussed.

REFERENCES

American Association of Colleges of Nursing, (1998). *The essentials of baccalaureate education for professional nursing practice*. Washington, DC: Author.

Boyd, E., & Fales, A. (1983). Reflective learning: Key to learning from experience. *Journal of Humanistic Psychology, 23*(2), 99–117.

Brown, H., & Sorrell, J. (1993). Use of clinical journals to enhance critical thinking. *Nurse Educator, 18*(5), 16–19.

Callister, L. (1993). The use of student journals in nursing education: Making meaning out of clinical experience. *Journal of Nursing Education, 32*(4), 185–186.

Cary, L. (1991). *Black ice*. New York: Random House.

Coles, R. (1993). *The call of service: A witness to idealism*. Boston: Houghton Mifflin.

Darbyshire, P. (1995). Lessons from literature: Caring, interpretation, and dialogue. *Journal of Nursing Education, 34*(5), 211–216.

Facione, N., & Facione, P. (1996). Externalizing the critical thinking in knowledge development and clinical judgment. *Nursing Outlook, 44*(3), 129–136.

Goldsmith, S. (1995). *Journal reflection: A resource guide for community service leaders and educators engaged in service learning*. Washington, DC: American Alliance for Rights & Responsibilities.

Gordon, R. (1994). Keeping students at the center: Portfolio assessment at the college level. *The Journal of Experiential Education, 17*(1), 23–27.

Gordon, R., & Julius, T. (1995). At the heart of education: Portfolios as a learning tool. In B. Horwood (Ed.), *Experience and the curriculum* (pp. 93–109). Dubuque, IA: Kendall/Hunt.

Hahnemann, B. (1986). Journal writing: A key to promoting critical thinking in nursing students. *Journal of Nursing Education, 25*(5), 213–215.

Hansberry, L. (1969). *To be young, gifted and black.* New York: Random House.

Horwood, B. (Ed.). (1995). *Experience and the curriculum.* Dubuque, IA: Kendall/Hunt.

Jacoby, B. (1996). *Service-learning in higher education.* San Francisco: Jossey-Bass.

Joseph, J. (1994). *When I am an old woman I shall wear purple* (2nd ed.). New York: Sidney and Doubleday.

Kirkpatrick, M. (1994). NINE Newspapers in nursing education. *Nurse Educator, 19*(6), 21–23.

Kolb, D. (1984). *Experiential learning: Experience as the source of learning and development.* Englewood Cliff, NJ: Prentice-Hall.

Krueger, R. (1988). *Focus groups: A practical guide for applied research.* Newbury Park, CA: Sage.

Lame Deer, J., & Erdoes, R. (1972). *Lame Deer: Seeker of visions.* New York: Simon & Schuster.

Mezirow, J. & Associates (1990). *Fostering critical reflection in adulthood: A guide to transformative and emancipatory learning.* San Francisco: Jossey-Bass.

Mezirow, J. (1991). *Transformative dimensions of adult learning.* San Francisco: Jossey-Bass.

Morgan, D. (1997). *Focus groups as qualitative research* (2nd ed.). (Qualitative Research Methods Series, Vol 16). Thousand Oaks, CA: Sage.

National League for Nursing Accrediting Commission. (1996). *Criteria and guidelines for the evaluation of baccalaureate and higher degree programs in nursing.* New York: National League for Nursing Press.

Rodriguez, R. (1992). *Days of obligation: An argument with my Mexican father.* New York: Penguin.

Santiago, E. (1993). *When I was Puerto Rican.* New York: Random House.

Saylor, C. R. (1990). Reflection and professional education: Art, science and competency. *Nurse Educator, 15*(2), 8–11.

Schon, D. A. (1983). *The reflective practitioner: How professionals think in action.* New York: Basic Books.

Sedlak, C. (1997). Critical thinking of beginning baccalaureate nursing students during the first clinical nursing course. *Journal of Nursing Education, 36*(1), 11–18.

Silcox, H. (1995). *A how to guide to reflection: Adding cognitive learning to community service programs.* Holland, PA: Brighton Press.

Stevens, P. (1996). Focus groups: Collecting aggregate-level data to understand community health phenomena. *Public Health Nursing, 13*(3), 170–176.

Valiga, T., & Bruderle, E. (1997). *Using the arts and humanities to teach nursing: A creative approach.* New York: Springer Publishing Company.

Wong, F., Kember, D., Chung, L., & Yan, L. (1995). Assessing the level of student reflection from reflective journals. *Journal of Advanced Nursing, 22,* 48–57.

CHAPTER 4

The Promises and Problems of Service-Learning

Dona Rinaldi Carpenter, Ed.D., R.N., C.S., & Patricia Harrington, Ed.D., R.N.

> Hundreds of thousands of us will be faced with a great emptiness...unless our education and experiences are not only on-going but on-giving.
>
> —*Alec Dickson*

A well-established service-learning program can bring with it many positive experiences for those involved. The foundation has been laid in the preceding chapters for establishing a service-learning program, integrating service into the curriculum, and strategies for reflection. Chapter Four summarizes the promises of service-learning and examines some of the problems that may arise along with possible solutions. Most importantly, the reader will see that the promises of service-learning far outweigh the problems, and the problems . . . really are not problems. Rather, the "problems" associated with a service-learning program are better described as "stumbling blocks" which might be avoided. Ultimately, the success of any service-learning program lies in the commitment and leadership of the faculty involved. Addressing problems up front, as in any other teaching situation, will eliminate complications and contribute to the development of a sound and successful program.

THE PROMISES OF SERVICE-LEARNING

The promises of integrating service-learning into the nursing curriculum should be quite evident to the reader at this point in the text. Once convinced of the connection between service and learning it can be difficult to imagine why one would not incorporate this type of teaching pedagogy. The benefits to the education of students can be seen in the examples that have been provided. The reader is reminded, however, that what students learn and how they grow through the service-learning experience will vary from one institution to the next.

Clearly, there are certain expectations for all service-learning programs that will be similar across states and across the nation. These expectations have been identified by the International Partnership for Service-Learning. The International Partnership for Service-Learning is an incorporated not-for-profit consortium of colleges, universities, service agencies, and related organizations united to foster and develop programs linking community service and academic study. (See Appendix A: Resources). The Partnership holds that the joining of study and service:

- is a powerful means of learning;
- addresses human needs that would otherwise remain unmet;
- promotes intercultural/international literacy;
- advances the personal growth of students as members of the community;
- gives expression to the obligation of public and community service by educated people; and
- sets academic institutions in right relationship to the larger society

All service-learning programs should expect to see positive growth in the areas identified by the partnership, while specific experiences will be individualized and different for every student, faculty member, and institution. The expectations identified by the International Partnership for Service-Learning programs, and how they become a reality, have been highlighted throughout this book. They can be viewed as the capstone expectations for any solid service-learning program.

Another way to look at the promises of service-learning is through an illustration involving questions and answers, as well as the voices of students who have lived the experience. In an article by Wills (1992) the following questions were posed for the reader to consider with regard to service- learning:

Why should colleges and universities engage in service and service-learning? What is to be gained? Don't such activities detract from the real rigors of education, which many believe should be confined to the classroom or the library or the laboratory? Isn't there a time for service and a separate time for learning? (p. 35).

Having reached this point in this book, the reader can probably answer these questions with some sense of conviction. The answers to the questions offered by Wills (1992) might include:

"Why should colleges and universities engage in service and service-learning?" (Wills, 1992, p. 35). Colleges and universities should engage in service-learning to broaden the scope of classroom content; provide exposure to and awareness of the needs of the surrounding community; enhance students' critical thinking abilities; develop leadership skills; and instill in our future leaders a sense of responsibility in terms of giving back to the communities in which they live. This is certainly not a complete list of reasons to engage students in service-learning, but is absolutely a place to begin. In the words of one student:

I feel that learning in the community impacts my academic life here at the University. While I was working I learned more about what kind of person I am and more about others. I don't think that I realized this as much before I started volunteering. This has also affected my academic life. I now think about other things in life besides my studies, which has resulted in less stress. I am receiving higher grades now, which could be because of the fact that I am not as stressed as last semester. I believe that only good things come out of service-learning. Through this program both the student and the community benefit.

"What is to be gained?" (Wills, 1992, p. 35). What will be gained from engaging students in a solid service-learning experience is in many ways an unknown. Surely, an increased sensitization to the needs of the communities and a broader exposure and application to theoretical issues will occur. But each student, each faculty member, and each recipient in the service-learning experience will walk away with a new way to view the world and a new understanding of the needs of others. Their experiences will be and should be unique.

Berry (1995) emphasized that:

> We need to keep in mind the powerful transformative dimension of ser-vice-learning. Open-ended service-learning allows students the freedom to find their own values. Imposing pre-set agendas may also work against the often-stated desire to have service-learning become part of the mainstream of education. Setting a priori learning and values agen-das is a sure way to alienate faculty (p. 4).

Finally, Berry (1995) notes:

> Students should be allowed to move beyond simplistic answers and come to their own conclusions about the complexity of social, cultural and international issues. Establishing preconceived agendas for devel-opmental and learning outcomes is to turn the value and importance of service-learning, intellectual growth, values development and indeed, education itself, on its head." (p. 4).

What is to be gained from service-learning can also be heard in the voices of students:

> I fulfilled my service-learning at the Boys and Girls Club of America. Here I was granted the opportunity to interact with the socially and eco-nomically deprived children of the community, which was quite an expe-rience. Despite my own original, personal shortcomings with regard to working with children in this young age group, I found myself gradually growing as an individual. With each visit I made to the club, I was learn-ing more and more about the person I was. Yet, even more importantly, I was discovering the potential that I possessed inside to become the per-son that I wanted to be. As ironic as it may seem, I feel that I learned more from the children themselves than they did from me.

"Don't such activities detract from the real rigors of education, which many believe should be confined to the classroom or the library or the lab-oratory?" (Wills, 1992, p. 35). Service-learning experiences that are well designed do not detract from, but rather add to the rigors of education. Nursing, in particular is very familiar with the important learning that takes place in the clinical setting for students. Without this experiential type of learning, what is transmitted in the classroom may never have any real meaning for the student. For example, one can explain the signs and symptoms of hypoglycemia to a student in the classroom setting, but until the student actually experiences the care involved for a patient with this problem, the theoretical discussion will not have the same meaning. Service-learning, in similar, yet different ways, brings new meaning to the theory presented in the classroom situation. Through reflection, journaling activities, and papers, service-learning adds to the rigors of the classroom. Opportunities for faculty and students to engage in service-based research projects complements learning and has potential to enhance faculty scholarship. Again, the students tell the story best:

> Learning in the community through service-learning is a good experience. It helped me to see what I liked and what I thought I could be good at. Service-learning impacts academic life because you are learning things outside of the classroom, about things that you can't learn in a room while the teacher lectures. Your academic life is enhanced because the experiences make you more interested in the subject matter. Learning things in class and then seeing the theory in practice provides experiences that make the service-learning requirement worthwhile.

"Isn't there a time for service and a separate time for learning? (Wills, 1992, p. 35). Service and learning must be viewed as inseparable concepts if the program is truly service-learning. Certainly, one can learn in the classroom setting, and one can learn in the service setting. But when the experiences are interrelated and used to stimulate class discussion regarding critical social issues and community needs, the learning is inseparable. The understanding of theory now depends on the experiences gained in the service setting, and the service setting experience is related to the theory presented in the classroom situation. As one student wrote:

> My service-learning experience helped me in ways that I could not even begin to count. It not only made me aware of the work of a hospital, it made me realize that someday I will be the nurse in charge and I need to strive to be the best nurse I can be.

The promises that a solid service-learning experience can bring to the education of students has been discussed throughout this text and can be seen in the answers that might be provided to the questions asked by Wills (1992) as well as comments made by students involved in service-learning experiences. Personal and professional growth beyond what one could ever expect in the classroom setting can occur when there is a well-organized program that is grounded in faculty leadership and strong administrative support. The preparation required before initiating such endeavors is time-consuming and detailed. Not only does the service-learning component need to be developed and integrated, but faculty and students need to change the way they teach and learn. As Leder and McGuinness (1996) have emphasized:

> Service learning is not a simple add-on ("oh yes, and spend a morning in the soup-kitchen"); rather, it challenges one to rethink the texts read, as well as the modes of discussion, writing, and testing employed in the classroom. In addition, faculty may encounter increased personal burdens. Suddenly, there are demands to help student liaisons with service sites, and to address the practical or emotional problems that arise there (p. 48).

A service-learning program requires planning, faculty commitment, administrative support, and ongoing follow-up and evaluation. Without a firm commitment from the faculty and administration to develop a service-learning program, there will be more obstacles and opportunity for failure.

Clearly, service-learning as a pedagogical method has very substantial benefits that will contribute to the education of all those involved. In addition to promoting student awareness of the needs of people from diverse backgrounds and age groups, service-learning has added benefits for nursing faculty and for the college or university. Personal experiences with service-learning can provide faculty with a deeper appreciation of the importance of a community-based curriculum. With new awareness of community needs, faculty can proceed with curriculum revisions to include community experiences that are not mere "add-ons". Rather, service experiences will be based on knowledge of the community's needs. The relationships developed with community partners will serve to enhance students' experiences in the future.

For example, students and faculty participated in HIV women's' outreach with the American Red Cross. While working with women in subsidized housing developments, they became aware of other additional health-promotion needs of this particular population. As a result of this experience, plans are underway to establish a permanent "clinical group" at the housing development. Students will provide health promotion programs on hypertension, breast self-exam, and other issues identified by the residents.

Another benefit to faculty is an opportunity to participate in service-generated research. Effective planning for service-learning in each course should consider faculty research interests and attempt to connect service opportunities with community settings that match faculty interests. In this way, faculty enthusiasm for service-learning will be connected to research and teaching agendas, and ultimately will be viewed more positively by faculty.

The benefits to the department of nursing and to the university will be substantial, and include increased visibility in the local media and opportunities to collaborate with colleagues at other colleges and universities. For example, in a recent article in the local newspaper about hospice services in Northeastern Pennsylvania, comments by nursing students involved in service-learning at the University of Scranton were highlighted. Agency partners have also included articles about students in their newsletters. In fact, the American Red Cross highlights our collaborative HIV Prevention Program in their *National Resource Directory on Young Adult Volunteer Programs*. Success with service-learning has stimulated the interest of nursing colleagues in the region, who look to the program described for guidance as they prepare to institute service-learning in their nursing programs. Two collaborative projects have emerged from this interest.

A well grounded service-learning program may be one of a student's most meaningful experiences, and an experience that cannot be obtained in any other way. A connection between academic study and broader social issues can be made and developed into a lifelong opportunity for service to society. Such programs, however are not without their problems. Some of the issues and problems that may arise related to service-learning programs follow.

PROBLEMS OF SERVICE LEARNING

The problems associated with service-learning are really more stumbling blocks than actual problems. Careful planning and coordination can prevent some of the pitfalls that are addressed in the following pages. Issues that need careful consideration include: coordination and support for the service-learning program; developing faculty commitment and leadership; evaluation and follow-up; and legal liability and safety issues.

Coordination and Support

Before one can even begin to think about initiating a service-learning program, issues related to coordination and support must be addressed. Faculty, administration, and students must be informed and supportive of service-learning if such a program is to succeed.

Faculty are the key to the start of a successful service-learning program. Therefore, faculty must be informed and committed to the program development before planning is initiated. Nursing faculty are familiar with many of the activities associated with service-learning and therefore the concepts of reflection, journaling, and community service are not as difficult to master as they might be for faculty from disciplines where these pedagogical methods are not widely used. Orientation programs and reading the literature related to service-learning is a good place to begin once faculty have agreed to examine the concept. Financial support for faculty to attend national conferences on incorporating service-learning in the curriculum, and developing skills in critical reflection, are important for success. Matching faculty expertise and research interests with the types of service provided can facilitate program development. An academic-community partnership described by Maurana and Goldenberg (1996) suggested other faculty rewards, including "assistance with article publication, and recognition and awards for innovative education at both school and university levels"(p. 429).

Administrative support is also essential. Service-learning programs require supportive personnel to work with faculty. These individuals may come in the form of graduate assistants, secretarial support, or help from a volunteer office on campus. This support, however, reconnects us to a concept presented in Chapter One. The university must have, as its mission, service to the larger community. If support begins at the mission level, then it can filter through the administration, to the faculty, and to the students.

Student commitment to service-learning emerges quickly. As freshmen, they enter the University with grand ambitions to serve others as professional nurses. As mentioned in earlier chapters, many students have had service experiences in high school and are eager to continue serving in the community. Some may even select a particular university because of the opportunities to engage in service. Incorporating service-learning into the freshman year is an important step to gain student support and enthusiasm for the program.

Developing Faculty Commitment and Leadership

In terms of the academic setting, issues related to promotion, tenure, and time constraints may emerge for faculty. The three cornerstones of faculty evaluation for promotion and tenure are research, teaching, and service. For nursing faculty, teaching loads may already be cumbersome, given the amount of time required to prepare and teach a clinical course. For example, if a faculty member is teaching a clinical rotation, this may involve 2 full days per week at a local hospital, working with students caring for multiple groups of patients. The clinical time each week may involve 16 intense hours, and consideration must then be given to the amount of time it takes to prepare the assignment and review prior to the actual experience. Often this is only part of the faculty load which is compounded by teaching a theory component, service, and research activities, not to mention faculty clinical practice. If faculty are concerned about promotion and tenure issues, they may be hesitant to try a new teaching pedagogy that might interfere with research time or perhaps have an adverse impact on their teaching evaluations. As Will (1992) notes, "Most institutions give teaching and research an importance that make service look like the weak sibling" (p. 32). Therefore, the connection of service to learning in the academic setting is critical if service-learning programs are to be seen as a valuable component to the academic preparation of students, and worthy of faculty commitment.

Faculty who are involved but not well-prepared or supportive of service-learning can contribute to the program's downfall. Faculty support and direction is imperative if students are to see the relevance of their service-learning experience to their academic education. It is in the classroom that the experiences encountered in the community can be turned into those "teachable moments" mentioned in Chapter One, "The survival of service as an important component of contemporary higher education is by no means assured. The single most important variable is faculty participation" (Zlotkowski, 1996, p. 22).

Coordinating a service-learning program means that someone needs release time to successfully manage the day-to-day operations. Archer (1996) offered the following comment related to coordinating a service-learning program:

There were many challenges, both programmatic and personal. First, was
the overall development of the program while simultaneously managing
the volunteers and sites. I wanted all involved, from the advisory board
to the volunteers, to feel ownership of the program" (p. 421).

Time constraints on faculty can be significant. Faculty must be involved
with, or at least very familiar with, the work of the agency. In the best of
all possible worlds, the faculty member would also volunteer at the agency
(Porter & Schwartz, 1993). Knowing the mission of the agency, the staff,
and the type of situations that students may encounter will enable the faculty member to assist students to maximize their experiences, and works
smoothly if students are assigned to one or two agencies. When students
in one class are serving at many agencies, this task becomes overwhelming for faculty, and support is critical. At the University of Scranton, this
problem is ameliorated with support from the Collegiate Volunteers Office,
whose staff are familiar with many agencies, and coordinate student placement along with the faculty. Other examples of support for faculty include
graduate assistants who read and respond to journals and coordinate student placements, or trained program assistants who can mentor students
(Hondagneu-Sotelo & Raskoff, 1994).

Another source of support to ease the constraints on faculty time are the
community agency partners. There will be times when service activities
evoke emotional issues that may be difficult for students to handle alone.
During these times, the skilled agency personnel can be valuable in assisting students to understand stressful situations. For example, in the hospice
setting, there is support for volunteers who work with death and dying
issues. However, this is not always the case at every agency, and unex-
pected events can occur. Several students at our university who worked
with school-aged children experienced some emotional strain in situations
where the children were not dressed appropriately for cold weather, or
needed money for a snack because they had not eaten all day. In several
instances, students reported, through journals, that they were giving money
to the children, and wanted to walk them home because, in one case, a
mother couldn't pick up her six-year-old son because "her nails were
wet!" Clearly, support for students to navigate emotional issues is a critical component that can be provided by agency staff and through journal
follow-up.

Besides the obvious emotional issues that can arise from the service-
learning experiences, students may encounter unfamiliar or hidden preju-

dices and stereotypes. Through journal feedback, faculty can help students handle situations that may reinforce negative stereotypes. Hondagneu-Sotelo and Raskoff (1994) caution that it is important to challenge stereotypes, and they suggest a comprehensive orientation on diversity that is reinforced in the course lectures. Collaboration between the service-learning coordinator and the cultural diversity group on campus to prepare students for diversity issues, as described by Zlotkowski (1996), may help to prevent negative stereotyping.

Evaluation and Follow-up

Connecting service to learning requires that it be based on course objectives, meet identified community needs, and provide opportunities for reflection about the service. In service-learning courses at the University of Scranton, a portion of the course grade is designated for service-learning activities. As Mohan (1995) points out, faculty may be concerned about giving academic credit for service, and methods to evaluate the effect of the service on the student are in need of further development. The authors found a tendency for grade inflation following the introduction of service-learning. In general, the grades are one-half a grade higher than they were before service-learning was required. For example, a student who might earn a grade of "B" in the course, would now earn a "B+". Usually between 5 and 15% of the course grade is based on service requirements. If students complete the required service hours, journals, and reflection, they receive full credit. Careful placement of service-learning in nursing courses will insure that grade inflation does not prevent identification of weak students who may not be able to master the nursing content.

Certainly the overall program goal that service-learning will lead to a life-long commitment to community service in the student must be examined. A follow-up survey of nursing graduates is one method used to evaluate this goal. Incorporating several questions about the effect of service-learning experiences on the graduates' career choices and their commitment to life-long service will help to identify whether this goal has been met. Including several questions about service-learning on 1-year and 3-year graduate surveys contributes to the evaluation process. At this time, there are indications that service is influencing students' career choices, as several students reflected:

This service experience has helped me to make the decision that I would like to work with kids in the future; this experience has taught me many things about myself; I think that I would really like to work with children when I graduate from college.

The service experience has changed my focus in nursing, I really want to work with the elderly now.

Service-learning cannot occur in a vacuum, and random acts of volunteering, although important, are not service-learning. Identification of community needs and the establishment of strong connections between the college or university and the community setting are imperative to the success of the program. Chapter Five provides the reader with narrative examples of three community agencies that emphasize the importance of these strong connections.

Involving community partners in reflection sessions for the purpose of maintaining strong connections and ongoing evaluation can be difficult. Time constraints imposed by work schedules and personal commitments can make it difficult for agency representatives to "escape" for a few hours. Therefore, it is important to ensure that time is not wasted, that there is a clear agenda that moves forward and stays on time, and that there is meaningful work accomplished in as few meetings as possible.

Follow-up with the agencies that students are serving is vital to the overall success of the program. Clearly, faculty do not want to send students to places where they are not welcome or needed and faculty need to know that the students are doing a responsible job in the service setting. Feedback from agency partners has been collected using focus group methodology at the end of each academic year. Evaluations from the past 3 years produced interesting and important information that was used to revised and improve the program. Aspects of service-learning that were identified included the need to 1) provide an orientation period at each agency; 2) encourage students to commit to serving an agency over several semesters; and 3) to conduct annual focus groups that provide the agency partners with an opportunity to contribute to the program evaluation.

The academic calendar can also present a problem for community agencies who come to rely on the service of students. Summer, winter, and holiday breaks leave a void in many agencies that is difficult to cope with. At the University of Scranton, we are examining ways to alleviate this "loss of service" for our agency partners. One possibility is to include service-learning in summer courses, or request volunteers through the Collegiate Volunteer Office to serve at the agencies for the summer and break periods.

Legal and Liability Issues

The area of legal and liability issues is another concern for universities implementing service-learning programs. Our duty to provide students with a safe learning environment is clearly spelled out in existing guidelines for safety on campus, including laboratory safety, hospital policies for students in the clinical setting, and travel risks for nursing students. Universities evaluate insurance policies regularly to assure that students are protected; yet, several questions remain difficult to answer. What about the service environment? Is the neighborhood that the agency is located in a safe place for students? Are the clients served at the agency a risk to students? Students in service-learning experiences have been placed in prisons, homeless shelters, and housing developments that are known to have high crime rates. The question remains, how can we protect students?

Porter and Schwartz (1993) made several suggestions to provide a safe environment for student service; "The faculty member . . . stressed safety precautions and appropriate student conduct both inside and outside the agency, not only with the class but also with the agency, the college administration, and the college legal counsel" (p. 413). The safety of those served is an issue that may be covered by community agency policies, such as feeding residents in a nursing home, transporting patients in a hospital, or playing with children in day-care and after-school centers. When the service ventures out into the community in the form of outreach efforts, going door-to-door with prevention information, the question must be asked: Who is liable if someone is injured? This is a grey area that bears investigation before service-learning is implemented, and campus volunteer offices or legal counsel may be able to provide some answers.

SUMMARY

Howard Berry (1995) notes that the "achievement of visibility and popularity carries consequences" (p. 3). He further elaborates:

> As the historian Herbert Muller has observed about organizations and movements which reach a certain point in their development: "Nothing

fails like success." Service-learning, particularly in higher education, stands poised at such a turning point, one which may well determine whether it takes its place as a foundational part of the mainstream of education and student development, or will join other education fads on the periphery (Berry, 1995, p. 3)

Service-learning programs will only continue to grow and develop if they are fully supported by faculty and administration. Otherwise they may very well disappear again, just as they did in the late 1970s. In this chapter we have presented the promises and problems of service-learning. With first-hand experiences to guide us, possible solutions to the problems have been suggested. Each program will be different in terms of promises and problems. Coordination and support, along with faculty commitment, will be essential. Most importantly, from the authors' perspectives, the promises have far outweighed the problems. Service-learning has clearly been worth the effort. In Chapter Five, the views of our community partners are presented.

REFERENCES

Archer, D. (1996) The community health advocacy program: Changing the relations between communities and the medical campus. *Medicine and Health, 79*(12), 420–421.

Berry, H. A. (1995). If I had a hammer . . . *Action/Reflection: The Partnership for Service Learning*, Winter, 3–4.

Hondagneu-Sotelo, P., & Raskoff, S. (1994). Community service-learning: Promises and problems. *Teaching Sociology, 22*, 248–254.

Leder, D., & McGuinness, I. (1996). Making the paradigm shift: Service learning in higher education. *Metropolitan Universities* 47–53.

Maurana, C. A., & Goldenberg, K. (1996). A successful academic-community partnership to improve the public's health. *Academic Medicine, 71*(5), 425–431.

Mohan, J. (1995). Thinking local: Service-learning, education for citizenship and geography. *Journal of Geography in Higher Education, 19*(2), 129–142.

Porter, J. R., & Schwartz, L. B. (1993). Experiential service-based learning: An integrated HIV/AIDS education model for college campuses. *Teaching Sociology, 21*, 409–415.

Wills, J. R. (1992). Service: On campus and in the curriculum. *Education Record*, 32–36.

Zlotkowski, E. (1996). A new voice at the table? Linking service-learning and the academy. *Change*, 20–27.

Community Partnerships in Service-Learning

Patricia A. Bailey, Ed.D., R.N., C.S.

> I am convinced that my life belongs to the whole community; and as long as I live it is my privilege to do for it whatever I can.
>
> —*George Bernard Shaw*

The building of community partnerships is an essential component of a successful service-learning program for any university. These partnerships cannot be established overnight, but require thoughtful exploration and mutual dialogue between the academic institution and targeted community sites. We must keep in mind that there needs to be a "fit" between academia and community, and both will need to focus on seeing their institutions as woven together rather than as being on opposite sides of a fence if there is to be a successful and sustained service-learning program. For a partnership to exist, the goals and objectives of both institutions must find common ground on which to build a stable service program.

Chapter Five describes essential elements of building community partnerships, discusses models of community partnerships, and gives three examples of how community partners view their relationship with the academic university.

STRENGTHENING COMMUNITY TIES

As one begins to explore partnerships with the community, certain criteria will support strong relationships. Both the university and the community should benefit from the partnership; the relationship should serve to support and strengthen the mission and goals of each institution. Each partner should be able to identify and reaffirm the supporting rationale for the partnership. There are many examples in the literature of successful academic-community partnerships focused on improving health. Maurana and Goldenberg (1996) describe a partnership between two academic institutions and a variety of individuals and agencies from a surrounding community. Known as the Center for Healthy Communities, it was formally institutionalized in 1994 in Dayton, Ohio. The authors stress the importance of ensuring that the community decides what their health issues and problems are, academic institutions can then enter into the partnership to assist and facilitate change within that community. The stress is on "doing with" the community and not "doing for" or "doing to" (p. 426).

Three essential principles for a successful community-academic partnership are described as: leadership, where trust is built and respect is shared as each strive toward a common mission; partnership, where teamwork is enhanced through open communication and sharing of resources; and empowerment, where all members of academia and community are strengthened in their self-determination and skill acquisition (Maurana & Goldenberg, 1996).

Cauley, Maurana, and Clark (1996), also involved in the Center for Healthy Communities, describe a community-academic partnership where both faculty and agency staff composed learning objectives for health professions students.

> This model, which involves more coordination and enhancing of existing resources, than it does creation of new services, is one that has implications for any system where service-learners abound and a community is ready to use their time and energy (p. 57).

Dilllon and Sternas (1997) define community empowerment as "the ability of the community to actively participate, through partnerships, in setting priorities for health care and implementing programs to promote health" (p. 2–3). Again, it is not "doing for" but "enabling to"!

Seifer, Connors, and O'Neil (1996) describe the goals of the Health

Professions Schools in Service to the Nation (HPSISN) program which focused on integration of service-learning into health professions courses and the development of community-campus partnerships that address unmet health needs.

A program for the incorporation of service-learning and community-oriented dental education (CODE) is described by Desjardins (1996). A major goal of this project was to "provide the opportunity to positively affect the values and attitudes of students toward community needs and access to care issues" (p. 822).

COMMUNITY-CAMPUS MODELS

There are various models of community relationships that can be utilized when planning for a service-learning program. Jacoby (1996) described three models: the clearinghouse model,where a central listing of available agencies is kept, and neither the university nor the community has a clear involvement in building a partnership; the partnership model, where both the university and the community join forces to establish a mutual and beneficial partnership to meet student and community needs, and is generally limited to a few specific agencies; and the collaboration model, where the university and the community work together on specific issues and the university actually assumes a role in addressing a community need, with student and faculty benefits becoming secondary. Based on the needs of the local community and the mission and goals of the university, one must decide which model is more appropriate or if a modified model will meet the needs of a particular program. At the University of Scranton, a modified program combining the clearinghouse/partnership model has been the framework for our service-learning program. A central Collegiate Volunteers Office on campus serves as a central point for connecting to a large listing of local community agencies. This office comes under the administration of the Vice-President for Campus Ministry and offers the following service-learning support:

- Provides up-to-date information on community needs and acts as liaison with agency personnel;
- Assists in the design and implementation of service-learning components into courses;

- Provides resource information on types of service experiences as they relate to a particular discipline;
- Assists in design and/or facilitation of a reflection component;
- Collects data on service-learning experiences from students, faculty, and community agencies; and
- Promotes awareness and understanding of service-learning in the university community through educational materials, training, and publicity.

At the University of Scranton, faculty utilized support from the Collegiate Volunteers Office in addition to establishing partnerships with specific community agencies such as the Jewish Home of Northeast Pennsylvania, the American Red Cross HIV/AIDS Education Program, and the Visiting Nurse Association Hospice Program. Again, the model for one's service-learning program must fit the uniqueness of each academic setting and local community.

Certain elements of program development can be added to help form and strengthen community partnerships. A Service-Learning Advisory Committee is a helpful first step in building community contacts. Members of such a committee could include key community agency personnel, university/department administrative staff, faculty, students, and any others essential to developing and advising a service-learning program. Advisory committees serve varied functions. They will advise and guide a program through development and continued evaluation. Membership can rotate as the need arises.

The use of focus groups also facilitates communication between the academic setting and the community agencies. These groups can meet on a yearly basis. With input from community partners, faculty, students, and administrative staff, the process of program evaluation and ongoing development can be enhanced. Conducting focus groups on and off campus is a great way to have community partners and academic personnel come together for genuine sharing and outcomes evaluation. Focus group goals need to be clearly outlined, and trained group facilitators should be responsible to lead the groups in discussion. In addition to advisory committees and focus groups, written materials for community partners are essential. Brochures and service-learning handbooks for community agencies are very helpful reference materials for agency personnel.

As we work at improving our programs, consistent communication with community staff is extremely important. Site visits to community programs, engaging community staff to assist with reflection times with students, and having community members present on the purpose and goals of their community organization to classes are all ways to foster strong community partnerships.

INTERGENERATIONAL SERVICE-LEARNING PROJECTS

The Nursing Department at the University of Scranton has worked to strengthen a number of community partnerships over the 3-year period of our HPSISN program grant. Three of these partners are the VNA Hospice of Lackawanna County, the Jewish Home of Northeastern Pennsylvania, and the American Red Cross of Scranton and Wyoming Valley. The following pages describe their stories.

VISITING NURSE ASSOCIATION HOSPICE OF
LACKAWANNA COUNTY
301 DELAWARE STREET
OLYPHANT, PA 18447
PEGGY BEGLEY, VOLUNTEER DIRECTOR

The VNA Hospice of Lackawanna County was established in 1989 as part of the original Visiting Nurse Association that has served our community since 1898. Hospice is specialized care that tends to the physical, emotional, social, and spiritual needs of seriously and terminally ill patients and their families.

Hospice care traditionally has centered around care of the terminally ill patients in their homes, as well as in nursing homes (which is their residence). There are times, however, when the patient may require inpatient care. VNA Hospice saw the need for an inpatient facility in the Scranton area, and in June of 1997 opened an 11-bed unit which consists of seven private and two semi-private rooms at Community Medical Center in Scranton. Our inpatient unit has been designed to provide the patient with a homelike environment with unlimited and unrestricted visiting hours, a gathering room equipped with a kitchenette for families to prepare special meals for patients if they wish, or a place for families to eat together in a warm atmosphere. The unit also includes a play area for our younger visitors, and laundry facilities and overnight accommodations for those family members who wish to spend the night. We are staffed with a hospice team of medical directors, nurses, social workers, counselors, certified nursing assistants, therapists, and volunteers who deliver the specialized care that the terminally ill and their families require.

The association between the VNA Hospice and the University of Scranton actually precede the hospice program of the Visiting Nurse Association. The Director of Hospice Services and the Volunteer Coordinator, were graduates of the University of Scranton. They were very aware of the giving nature of the students and faculty and wanted to build the volunteer program from that setting.

In 1989 the management team was invited to develop the VNA Hospice program, and shortly after opening that program, the new directors attended the Volunteer Fair sponsored by the University of Scranton. This forum allowed local agencies to come to the campus and actively recruit volunteers for their organizations. However, at that time, the hospice philosophy was relatively new to the area and not readily understood by many, therefore the number of volunteers that were interested was minimal.

Over the years, the public has become more aware and better educated about hospice. The focus of hospice is not on death, but on living life to the fullest. The agency operates from a basic philosophy which affirms life and neither hastens nor postpones death; our focus of care is redirected from curative to palliative care, with emphasis on comfort and support to encourage the patients' participation in life until death occurs.

In 1995, with the assistance of the University of Scranton's Nursing Department, hospice staff focused on recruiting nursing students to their program. This relationship has proven to be very successful. Of 80 volunteers in the hospice program, 18 are University of Scranton students. The agency's goal is to recruit students in their freshman or sophomore years so that they may remain with us and grow in their development and skill. The 8-hour orientation takes place over a period of 4 weeks, and is conducted on campus for the nursing students. A great emphasis is placed on the orientation process so that the volunteers receive as much information as possible to enable them to feel a valued part of the hospice team. Our goal is to keep these volunteers as part of our team until they graduate.

The experience the students encounter has been very productive for many of them. They have given the VNA Hospice a great deal of positive feedback. They feel this is a great learning experience; they assist the nursing staff, provide companionship to both patients and their families, feed patients, and assist with clerical duties such as answering phones, faxing, and computer work. Because their patients have been certified to be terminally ill, hospice care has a different focus, concentrating on palliative care, and covering all areas of a person's life: physical, emotional, social, and spiritual. Although the students begin with little or no experience, they eventually become comfortable with their roles. As students recognize their strengths and weaknesses, they develop their own unique talents in hospice volunteerism.

Working with students provides many challenges for the Volunteer Coordinator. Many students do not have transportation, and scheduling must be arranged around their classes, work schedules, and social calendars. They also have many breaks during the year, such as Christmas vacation, spring break, and summer vacation. During breaks in the academic schedule, the students are truly missed.

Working with students provides many benefits to our agency. Their youthful enthusiasm is most beneficial to our patients and staff. Some of the student volunteers find the work challenging and have shown interest in becoming hospice nurses. Two of the nursing students are certified nursing assistants and have accepted positions as part-time certified nursing assistants with the agency. Through their experience of caring for hospice unit and homebound patients, the students both increase community awareness of our agency and promote the hospice philosophy.

The continued relationship between the VNA Hospice of Lackawanna County and the University of Scranton Nursing Department is a "win-win situation" for everyone involved. It is obvious that the patients and their families receive the most benefit because the student volunteers provide the extra attention that is so important in this critical time of the patient's life. The VNA Hospice benefits because the program and the caregiving is enhanced by the volunteers' generosity of time and energy. Finally, the University and the students benefit from the rewards received by helping those in need. Nursing students get first-hand knowledge of the hospice philosophy, which will benefit them immensely when they embark upon their nursing careers. VNA Hospice of Lackawanna County feels it is vitally important to continue to build and sustain this relationship in the coming years.

THE JEWISH HOME OF EASTERN PENNSYLVANIA
1101 VINE STREET
SCRANTON, PA 18510
JANET MOSKOVITZ, VOLUNTEER COORDINATOR

Mrs. Selma Stark, at a 1915 meeting of the South Side Ladies Aid Society in Scranton, Pennsylvania, suggested that an organization be founded to care for the orphaned and neglected children and homeless elderly persons for whom there were no organized services. They named the institution they founded the "Jewish Home for the Friendless."

The first resident of the Jewish Home was admitted in 1921 to the facility located in the Providence section of Scranton. After some years the Home discontinued serving children in favor of foster care programs and dropped the negative word "Friendless" from the name, substituting the geographical designation which finally became the Jewish Home of Eastern Pennsylvania. The Jewish Home outgrew its original site and in April, 1964, the Home moved into its present quarters which were specially designed to serve elderly people. Since that time, the building has been expanded and services and programs were expanded and improved.

Today the Jewish Home is a fully-licensed skilled-nursing facility providing high-quality elderly care. A non-profit organization, the Jewish Home is a six-story nursing complex accommodating 175 individuals. Among the many beneficial on-site services available for residents are a high ratio of staff to residents, medical care, the Harry and Jeanette Weinberg Alzheimer's Unit and Program, rehabilitative care, highest-quality dietary services, licensed Social Workers, recreational activities, religious services for all faiths, and the Adult Day Care Program. In addition, the Jewish Home's continuum of care includes Webster Towers apartments for independent living seniors and Elan Gardens, an assisted-living facility for elderly who are independent in spirit, but in need of daily assistance.

"Bashert" is a lovely Yiddish word meaning "destined" or "fated." Perhaps it was Bashert that the Jewish Home and the University of Scranton were brought together. At the time I became Volunteer Coordinator of the Jewish Home, a relationship already existed between the University of Scranton students and the Jewish Home, mainly because of the Home's convenient location near the University. Only a few students managed to find adequate time in their busy schedules to volunteer in a nursing home.

Learning that Pat Vaccaro was Director of Collegiate Volunteers, I realized that the University of Scranton considered volunteering by its students to be an important component of their education. Because many students live away from home, volunteering gave them an opportunity to meld into the community. I contacted Pat to remind her we were neighbors and updated the handbook on volunteer opportunities available to interested students. Students from the University began to trickle in to the Home, offering to volunteer their services.

The impetus for a phone call to me from Patricia A. Bailey, Ed.D, the nursing professor who became Director of the service-learning program in the Department of Nursing, was the combination of the Jewish Home's location near the University and its elderly residents being a good resource for nursing students. Dr. Bailey realized the purpose and objective of the Nursing Department's service-learning project would be in harmony with those of the Jewish Home. Accessible to walking students, a stop on the Smart-Ride Bus route, and with a facility dedicated to the unique needs of each resident, the opportunities to volunteer and learn about the geriatric population seemed ideal.

While many benefits could accrue for the students, improving the quality of life and protecting the welfare of Jewish Home residents are the staff's greatest priorities. Because a defining moment of disease or disability often causes a person to be admitted to a nursing home, the admission creates significant upheaval in their lives. Residents leave behind not just their homes, but their privacy, families, friends, and neighborhood to arrive in a public accommodation filled with strangers. There is a certain loss of independence, some financial insecurity, and a change in social status. Who better to understand those changes than university students, who have gone through the very same process of leaving the security of home to begin a new phase of their lives?

The Jewish Home and the University of Scranton focus on the whole person. We recognize that a resident's and a student's physical, spiritual, emotional, and social needs are interrelated. This holistic approach stresses that dealing with one set of needs requires attention to all. Intergenerational relationships that would meet others' needs became the goal of the service-learning experience for the Nursing Department as well as for the Jewish Home staff.

The nursing students are people whose creativity, flexibility, sensitivity, communication skills, enthusiasm, friendliness, and desire to help others could brighten our residents' days. The students need to feel useful, appreciated, a part of the community, and suitably trained, and placement in a position that takes full advantage of their skills and experience is very appropriate.

As I explain to every student during my orientation session with them, "My role as Volunteer Coordinator is to make this a positive experience for you and our residents! If I succeed, you will come here eagerly and willingly, year after year, possibly for more than your required hours, and the residents will benefit greatly."

Each nursing home resident is a distinct person, each with his or her own feelings, reactions, and ability to adjust to the new environment. A nursing student at a university has the same traits, and, as they reach out to each other, there is potential to draw from the other's strengths and life experiences. Residents may have outlived family and friends or live far away from those they love. Students, while longing to be independent, often feel homesick and lonely. Residents serve as surrogate grandparents and role models, as students offer a willing ear and an eagerness to hear time-worn tales.

While training the students as volunteers, I impress on them the residents' medical problems and emotional losses. Nursing students are particularly sensitive to these issues. The volunteers' roles are to help reaffirm the residents' sense of dignity and self-worth. The students learn that the elderly may be different, disoriented, dependent, and even difficult, but that they are still valuable human beings deserving respect and encouragement.

When I give the new volunteers their orientation, I suggest the many areas of volunteer opportunities: friendly visiting, feeding, assisting with bingo and other games, accompanying field trips, serving as wheelchair escorts or walking assistants, mail delivering, entertaining, sewing, shopping, decorating, doing computer work, and helping with arts and crafts. I ask for their input. Do they have any special skills they would like to share? Do they want to create a program? Do they want to include friends who do or do not have service-learning requirements? Unlike student volunteers from other disciplines, nursing students offer to feed residents unable to feed themselves. The opportunity to work on a nursing unit and be hands-on with people who are in need of their help is very inviting. Eager to learn from the nurses on the floor and anxious to earn immediate gratification and experience, nursing students fulfill the greatest need for volunteers in the Jewish Home.

When I interview students for task placement, I make a statement that always brings a smile and look of relief to their faces: "Come and go as your school schedule fits into the Jewish Home's schedule and chose any volunteer opportunity you like—I do not assign you to specific tasks or hours." Those words are magic to the ears of stressed students and they visibly relax before my eyes. The simple truth is—these students are busy!

Do I think that being forced to balance schoolwork, a social life, sleep, exercise, and possibly a job is difficult? I get exhausted simply thinking about their schedules. Therefore, what works best for all is to make volunteering relaxing—a break from the day's travails. Do I succeed? As I sign the service-learning time sheet for the students at the end of the semester, I always ask the same question, "How did it go?" The most common response—"It was fun!" Fun to volunteer in a nursing home? Fun to see old people in wheelchairs? Fun to hear the same old stories over and over again? Fun to help someone play bingo for a token prize? Yes, it was Fun! Because, as they volunteered, the students heard first-hand stories about World War I, about life before television when going to silent movies cost a dime, and what it was like to leave home and friends to come to a new country with a strange language many, many years ago. Most importantly, the student volunteers felt needed and accomplished. I saw students pulled out of their shell of shyness by talkative residents. I saw shy residents open up in the brightness of a young person's interest. I heard students express guilt about missing a bingo game because a term paper was due. I saw sadness on faces of students not remembered by a favorite resident and panic upon hearing a resident had been taken to the hospital. I saw pride on the face of a nursing student feeding a resident who ate their entire meal.

Students volunteering in a nursing home may be forced to think about the finality of life, sickness, and loss of control. They may worry about their own ultimate death, or those of loved ones. They may come to fear the ravages of a long life—sickness, dehabilitation, and loneliness. They may also learn the value of life, the impact of choices, the worth of relationships, and the importance of human contact.

I feel that the outcome of service-learning in nursing education will be to create better nurses who are better citizens. I think they will be more compassionate, see the patient as a whole person, and care about the quality of life and the dignity of the individual. If a student decides from this experience that geriatrics is difficult and depressing and looks to a different branch of nursing for personal satisfaction, what a valuable life choice volunteering will have created. The intentions of the University of Scranton students are honorable, and none have appeared at my door angry or complaining that service-learning is unfair or undesirable. They are simply struggling to find a place for it in a very busy semester.

My suggestions to them are to spread the required hours out over the semester, not waiting until the last minute, to chose a project that will be enjoyable, as well as a learning experience, and to reap satisfaction from the gift of their time.

My advice to other Volunteer Directors is to be flexible. To the community agency, the students are volunteers, and we are not always their priority. By making the students feel welcome and by not inflicting them with guilt over schedule changes, they will be eager to fulfill their obligation and even donate extra hours when they can.

When explaining service-learning requirements to nursing students, the following advice will endear them to Volunteer Directors:

- Call and make an appointment for an interview with the appropriate person.
- If unable to keep the appointment, call to change or cancel.
- Be prepared to express your interests and talents.
- Know your class and work schedules and important semester dates.
- Be open-minded and willing to forget stereotypes.
- Ask questions—be sure this volunteer opportunity is right for you.
- Be willing to learn and follow agency rules.
- Do not be afraid or embarrassed about saying it is not right for you.
- Live up to your commitment.
- SMILE!

The University of Scranton is challenged to help its students find a community agency that meets their needs so that volunteering is a positive learning experience. On-site visits, printed handouts from agencies, student volunteers speaking to new students, and agency representatives speaking in classes can help make choosing a volunteer location easier and the decision more productive. The Jewish Home has benefited greatly from "word of mouth" spread by students. Modern technology and public relations techniques aside, nothing sells like a student telling a friend or classmate it is fun to volunteer at the Jewish Home!

An interdisciplinary team approach to resident care helps to meet the needs of the elderly at the Jewish Home. The professional staff offers personalized and compassionate care and attention to all residents. The student volunteers are an integral component of the team, helping to supplement social and emotional needs. Service-learning students, therefore, enhance the quality of care given to our residents by connecting them to the community and by complementing the warm, personal, human touch provided by staff.

It is extremely important to remember that the service-learning component of a class means that students volunteer because they "have to." The successful volunteer program for all involved results when the students "want to." The age and life experiences of these students must be considered in the process. Their fears can be very real and appropriate. They want, and are entitled to, meaningful assignments and a voice in expressing personal feelings about situations they encounter. Some are afraid they will be burdened with a project they find uninteresting or that they are unprepared to perform. They fear making mistakes and being embarrassed. Like everyone, the students thrive with appreciative comments from staff, informative job training, and clearly defined goals. If recurrent feedback from students indicates that these needs are not being met, neither the community agency nor the University program benefits.

A great challenge faced by the Jewish Home is facing final exam week and the summer vacation without student volunteers. Intersession and summer students do not have a service-learning component in their classes and rarely volunteer. As the community agencies and those they serve rely on the students' enthusiasm and commitment over the year, their sudden departure, though forewarned, is anticipated and ultimately felt with a great sense of loss. As more departments of the University of Scranton require service-learning components as a course requirement, more community agencies will benefit from the students' presence and suffer their absence during holiday and summer vacations. Possible solutions for this problem would be to allow students to meet their requirements over the course of a calendar year, rather than school year, or to encourage day students living locally to participate during the off season.

The greatest weakness I found in the service-learning and nursing program was the lack of feedback I received from the students. Simply put, they got a grade, but I did not. As a member of the Advisory Committee of the Service-Learning program, I have attended frequent meetings during the last three years and was consistently updated on the work being done by the university faculty, and other community agencies. Frequent focus meetings were extremely beneficial to me because I learned I was not encountering any unusual problems and because the group, particularly the University students, often suggested worthwhile solutions for my concerns. However, I feel a significant void by not knowing what is said about the Jewish Home in the journals and evaluations written by student volunteers.

One proposed reflection session at the Home did not materialize due to difficulty coordinating students' schedules. Face-to-face conversations with student volunteers usually earn me two- or three-word answers to my queries about their experiences with residents; what they liked, hated, or felt uncomfortable about; and what I can do to improve our community-campus relationship. Common sense tells me it works, because I have students returning after their summer vacation, eager to renew relationships with residents. I feel, however, we would all benefit greatly if I could meet with "my" volunteers during their class time or reflections session and learn about their journal entries. Obviously, it would be easier for the agency representative to come to the students. I also believe the students have earned the "perk" of having the Volunteer Director join them at their convenience. I know the students would appreciate my interest, and I am convinced I would better serve the University of Scranton and the Jewish Home with the knowledge I gain from these informational gatherings.

I am honored to be a community partner of the service-learning and nursing program and I hope to continue to be a liaison between the University of Scranton and the Jewish Home for many years to come. It would be especially enlightening to have the students reflect on the volunteer experiences after they have been practicing nurses for a few years. Their observations on whether these requirements had an impact on their lives and careers would be fascinating, insightful, and informative to us all.

I personally believe it is a very important program for the University of Scranton and the Jewish Home and I have no doubt whatsoever that the world will benefit from the compassionate and competent nurses who have completed the service-learning project. The result has been a great benefit for some of those who need and deserve it most of all . . . Jewish Home residents.

AMERICAN RED CROSS
545 JEFFERSON AVENUE
SCRANTON, PA 18510
TRACY LYN SVALINA, DIRECTOR HEALTH SERVICES

Clara Barton founded the American Red Cross (ARC) on May 21, 1881. The mission of the ARC focuses on relief services to disaster victims and helping people prevent, prepare for, and respond to emergencies. Along with these disaster services, the ARC supplies blood to hospitals, provides CPR and first-aid Training, and in 1985 started educating the public about the HIV/AIDS epidemic. Clearly, all of the Red Cross programs depend on nurses, and Red Cross service opportunities are an excellent way to introduce nursing students to an organization that provides such an important service to society.

The collaboration between the Scranton Chapter of the American Red Cross and the University of Scranton Department of Nursing began in 1985, when a group of students and two faculty members were trained to take health histories and assess hemoglobin levels for campus and community blood drives. A strong partnership developed during the ensuing years as students served the chapter on numerous blood drives. During the 1980s, as the HIV epidemic spread across the country and the world, the need for HIV education became apparent and the American Red Cross HIV Education Program was established. Through posters, brochures, films, and public service announcements over television, and radio and in the press, tens of millions of Americans have been given a chance to learn the facts about HIV/AIDS.

When planning the service-learning program, nursing faculty identified community agencies that attracted students to service activities, and the Red Cross was one of them. In the service-learning program, students serve two Red Cross chapters. They serve the Scranton Chapter as HIV instructors in campus-based programs for their peers, and community-based programs for high school and junior high school students. Senior nursing students serve the Wyoming Valley Chapter as part of the Women's HIV Outreach Program.

In Chapter Two, the importance of faculty leadership was emphasized. The partnership with the Red Cross for HIV Peer education is an example of the benefits of faculty involvement in community service. Since 1992, two nursing faculty members, serving the Red Cross as HIV Instructor-Trainers, have provided the HIV Instructor Course to over 120 students (both nursing majors and non-nursing majors) and to 15 faculty and staff at the University of Scranton. Choosing the Red Cross as a partner in service-learning was beneficial, since a firm foundation for collaboration had already been established. The two aspects of student service in the HIV education program are described from the perspective of American Red Cross staff liaisons at each chapter, Scranton and Wyoming Valley.

When service-learning was initiated in 1995, nursing students were offered HIV instructor training. During the first year of the service-learning program, 14 students were certified as HIV instructors, and worked closely with the Scranton Chapter staff to present HIV prevention programs to high school and junior high school students. During the first year, the nursing students presented to a variety of young adult groups.

In one rural school district, the nursing students presented to an entire 7th-grade class. To facilitate the students' presentations in each class, the teacher left the room, providing the 7th graders with an opportunity to ask questions about HIV prevention that they may have felt uncomfortable asking if their teacher was in the classroom. At another school, the nursing students were part of a school-wide Health Fair, "Lifestyles: Know Your Risks" for high school juniors. The program met with tremendous success, and the students were invited back for a second presentation the following year. Four local high school programs were offered, and during eight sessions on HIV Prevention, the nursing students, along with the Red Cross staff were able to deliver the important message about HIV prevention to over 2,000 high school students.

During the second year of the service-learning program, nursing students assisted the Red Cross staff in conducting peer training for high school students. The university peer educators met with the high school peer educators, and discussed the problems they had encountered in presenting HIV information to college and high school students. The high school students respected the nursing students as role models, whose input was extremely valuable as they prepared to present HIV information.

Each chapter of the American Red Cross is expected to provide information on HIV/AIDS, helping to save lives by educating the public about this epidemic. The students who volunteer their time to do these presentations through the University of Scranton's service-learning program have assisted the Scranton Chapter in surpassing the expectations of its National Headquarters. Among the efforts of the staff, volunteers, and the university peers, the Scranton Chapter has been able to secure an "excellent" rating for HIV/AIDS community education for the past 3 years. The chapter has not only benefited by meeting its rating goal through its association with the peer educators, but they also have contributed so much more to the Red Cross. The peers possess an incredible amount of enthusiasm that is passed on to any audience they visit. This in turn makes the audience want to listen to the information that is shared. The age of the peers is another advantage. Most of the presentations that are done are aimed at the younger population, and the peers are young enough for the students to relate to, but are old enough for the students to look up to.

Working with the students' schedules can be difficult. They are usually in class when the high schools are in session. There is coordination on both the part of the peer and the middle school or high school requesting the presentation. Summer months, when the nursing students are not on campus, are not problematic because the public schools are not in session either. Transportation can be cause for concern because not all college students have cars. There is a van that the students can request to use to enable them to get to their service projects. One of the difficulties that many of the Red Cross's HIV Instructors face is the diversity of both the subject matter and the people who are receiving the information. Most of the college students fit a particular mold—they are from a White, middle-class household. It is difficult for many people to reach outside of what they know and try to connect with an individual who is different, either racially, ethnically, or culturally. There is diversity training within the Instructor course, but additional training could be used for all instructors.

Organizations always face minor trials when working with volunteer staff, but the amount of good, quality work that volunteers give to that organization far outweighs the stumbling blocks. The nursing students' commitment to HIV/AIDS education and the American Red Cross, and the commitment that the University has to the Scranton Chapter, is something that is extraordinary. The Scranton Chapter could not fulfill all of the requests for HIV/AIDS presentations without the students' participation. This past year the Scranton Chapter presented the HIV/AIDS Volunteer of the Year Award to the University of Scranton's Nursing Department and Wellness Center for all of their dedication in promoting the mission of the American Red Cross to educate the public about HIV/AIDS. We look forward to continuing our positive and productive partnership for many years to come!

WYOMING VALLEY CHAPTER AMERICAN RED CROSS
WOMEN'S OUTREACH PROGRAM
156 S. FRANKLIN ST.
WILKES-BARRE, PA. 18701
CANDAL B. SAKEVICH, WOMEN'S OUTREACH COORDINATOR

The American Red Cross has been providing HIV/AIDS education to the public since 1985. The Wyoming Valley Chapter is located in Wilkes-Barre, Pennsylvania, 15 miles south of the University of Scranton campus.

The Women's Outreach Program serves both Wilkes-Barre and Scranton. Ms. Candal Sakevich is the Women's Outreach Specialist, her partnership with senior nursing students is presented.

Through a grant from the Northeast Regional HIV/AIDS Coalition-Wyoming Valley United Way, the Wyoming Valley Chapter of the American Red Cross has been providing Women's Outreach since 1995 in a six-county region. Cases of AIDS in U.S. women have increased annually since the epidemic was first recognized in 1981. The purpose of Women's Outreach is to educate, promote healthy behavior change, and discuss harm reduction techniques with women, specifically economically disadvantaged women. Through Outreach services, women are given resource information and prevention materials that are needed to keep from becoming HIV-infected. Because the special needs of this population are so diverse, it is important to use a variety of teaching methods. Generally, when people think of education, they tend to imagine a structured, formal setting and curriculum. Outreach, much like service-learning, is based on concrete objectives, but is creative in its delivery of information.

When I became a Women's Outreach Specialist in July 1995, programs were offered to economically disadvantaged women who were enrolled in job training classes, were living in shelters, or were part of existing clubs or groups. Although the educational programs were based on The American Red Cross HIV/AIDS curriculum, the program format was adapted to the population of women who were served. Women were being reached, but often the educational contacts were a one-time occurrence. The need to expand the HIV/AIDS Outreach program was vitally necessary if changes in behaviors were to be accepted by the women. By using nontraditional forms of education, specifically short, repeated one-to-one contacts and informal small-group discussions, I was able to determine the needs of the women I served, while at the same time develop their trust. By working with the women, I helped them to become aware of their potential risk factors and identify various harm reduction techniques that were acceptable to them.

To perform this type of outreach, I literally walked through the public housing developments and approached the women who lived there. Since the women were on familiar ground, they were more willing to talk and listen. Because I represented the American Red Cross, women were more accepting of the information and would open up and ask questions. Through these contacts, I helped to empower women to teach their families and friends and protect themselves from HIV. I provided them with resource information, prevention materials, and age-appropriate literature for their children.

During the winter months of 1997, I was planning indoor outreach activities for the women in public housing. After discussing some of these ideas with a nursing faculty member from the University of Scranton, who was also a member of The Northeast Regional HIV/AIDS Planning Coalition, she informed me of the Service-Learning Program at The University of Scranton. The students who volunteered with the Women's Outreach Program were HIV/AIDS-certified instructors so they were already qualified to educate. I did want the students to understand some of the diversities of this group before they participated in the Outreach Program. In preparation, they met with the manager from one of the facilities, who talked openly and honestly of the situations many economically disadvantaged women find themselves in, including drug and alcohol abuse and domestic violence situations. In addition to this, I shared some of my outreach experiences with them. Basically, this population experiences every social problem imaginable. We, as Outreach workers, must tailor our programs according to those issues, while remaining nonjudgmental.

"Movie Night" was the first project the students worked on for Women's Outreach. This activity was designed to educate women regarding HIV by using a box-office movie to facilitate discussion. The next project was an activity night, addressing healthy behaviors for the children who lived in public housing. The nursing students taught the children how germs are spread and how handwashing can help them to stay healthy. Both the children and the students had an incredible chemistry together, and everyone had a great deal of fun. When the semester had ended, the students had completed their required number of service-learning hours, but still wanted to participate in one-to-one Outreach. I was extremely impressed with the willingness to sacrifice and the enthusiasm of these students. They were not "filling hours," they were serving the less fortunate of the community because they wanted to.

At this point, I had been providing Outreach services for 1 year in public housing. Since we wanted to measure the impact of Outreach and contact more residents, we went door-to-door with an oral pre- and post-test survey of HIV knowledge. We had permission from the Housing Authority to approach the residents in this way. By following both the University of Scranton's Institutional Review Board standards for protection of human subjects, and American Red Cross standards, we were careful to respect the residents' privacy. Any information collected was kept strictly confidential.

The degree of respect and compassion was obvious every time I saw the students talk and laugh with the women in the development. I saw shy and nervous students open up and engage strangers in meaningful dialogue. Residents whom I had never met before opened their doors and stopped to listen to the students and were interested in what they had to say.

Because the students were sensitive to the circumstances of the women and believed in the message they were giving, the picture was one of women helping women. There were no age, race or class barriers, just one person reaching out to another—"Outreach." The students were incredible to work with. Since they were trained in HIV education and were understanding of the diversities of the women, they met the needs of the Women's Outreach Program. By working with the students, I was able to contact more residents while maintaining quality outreach and meaningful dialogue. Any pitfalls such as scheduling and transportation were worked out by the students. Collectively, we agreed on the times to provide Outreach services and the students were there. After a long day in class or clinical, I am sure they were totally exhausted, but they barely showed any sign of it.

The greatest challenge was continuing the outreach program at its previously high standard after the students were gone. Unfortunately, the service-learning program is not implemented into the summer classes. When the students were gone, the impact was felt every time a resident or child asked: "Where's the girls?". If the students were able to complete the requirements over a 1-year time period, this problem might be eliminated. If service-learning were implemented into other disciplines, there would be summer classes that had this component.

One weakness I found with the service-learning program was the lack of feedback. The positive feedback I did receive was voluntary on behalf of the students and the Nursing Department. It would be beneficial to any agency to have a formal feedback or evaluation procedure. This would serve as a tool for growth for any agency.

Working with the University of Scranton nursing students has been a valuable experience for me, as I am sure it has been for them. However, there are some things I would do differently. I would make sure that I oriented the students to every facet of the agency because of the variety of services the Red Cross provides. I would also be sure to inform the students of our program evaluation procedures so that they will help us attain success. I would be sure to inform the students how and why we record demographics. Above all, I would develop an evaluation form for the students to complete about the Womens Outreach Program.

Overall, working with the University of Scranton Nursing Students and the Service-Learning Program has been of great benefit to me personally and to the agency, but most of all to the women we serve. Building a partnership through service-learning is a valuable endeavor that academic settings and Community agencies should consider!

SUSTAINING PARTNERSHIPS

As the above three stories indicate, sustaining partnerships takes planning, time commitments, a willingness to share in each other's mission, and a concern for enhancing students' learning and meeting the needs of a community. Our community partners have been in contact with the University regarding input of students and overall evaluation. This contact between the academic setting and the community is essential in sustaining partnerships. The focus-group sessions held each year with community members, faculty, and students has helped us in evaluating the needs of the community and how students are assisting in meeting those needs. These meetings have been very productive and have given us positive feedback on students' service. They have also assisted us in making changes in regard to advising and orienting students to a particular agency. Some comments from focus sessions with community members are:

- *Meet needs of the agency:* Nursing students help the residents one-on-one with enthusiasm and eagerness; they provide role models, friends, mentors, and tutors for the children; they go beyond the requirement and have great commitment.
- *Strengths:* Both the organization and the students benefit; give a youthful view of new ideas. A pool of work hours was guaranteed for some parts of the semester.
- *Weaknesses:* Summer and Intersession breaks; those who volunteer only to fulfill the requirement; erratic work performance.
- *Preparation needed:* Tour; an overview of the population students will be dealing with when they volunteer; know the agency's mission and role in the community or a "real-life view".
- *Expectation from students:* One hour a week with individual attention; be reliable, dependable, have the ability to listen and not push opinions; be there, and understand that service is more than just putting in time.

- *How to strengthen partnerships:* More feedback and better communication; include community in reflection activities; Keep focus groups—very positive for communication.

From reading these comments, it is easy to see how important interaction and communication with community partners is to sustaining a relationship that is beneficial to both the community and students. Opportunities to dialogue with community partners and problem-solve issues of student service have proven very valuable in regard to strengthening partnerships and improving the program. Engaging the community partners in an ongoing evaluation plan is essential for program development. Faculty need to decide on innovative ways to include key community agency personnel in the beginning development of a service-learning project. Whether this takes the form of having community representation on department committees or organizing an advisory committee consisting of community partners, faculty, and students, will depend on the individual program. The essential point here is that community partners need to be engaged in the process of developing a program from the very beginning. Then they need to be kept involved throughout the development and ongoing growth of the program. Just as a reciprocal relationship exists between what the students learn and what community needs are met, so too should a reciprocal relationship exist between the faculty planning for student learning needs and community personnel working to meet the needs of those in the community. We will continue to strive in the direction of improved communication with our community partners. Only then will the recipients of our service and our students realize the full benefit of service in the community and its impact on student learning and lifelong development!

SUMMARY

This chapter has examined the essentials of building community partnerships. Various models have been described, and three community partners have shared their thoughts and experiences regarding their own campus partnerships. Building and sustaining community partnerships requires a great deal of effort on the part of both the academic setting and the community agency. However, the benefits of such partnerships far outweigh the time and effort needed. Students and community recipients of service are all winners. It is well worth the effort!

REFERENCES

Cauley, K., Maurana, C., & Clark, M. (1996). Service-learning for health professions students in the community: Matching enthusiasm, talent, and time with experience, real need, and schedules. *Expanding Boundaries: Serving and Learning*, Corporation for National Service, January, 54–57.

Desjardins, P. (1996). Creating a community-oriented curriculum and culture: Lessons learned from the 1993–1996 ongoing New Jersey experiment. *Jounral of Dental Education, 60*, (10), 821–826.

Dillon, D., & Sternas, K. (1997). Designing a successful health fair to promote individual, family, and community health. *Journal of Community Health Nursing, 14*, (1), 1–14.

Jacoby, B. (1996). *Service-Learning in higher education.* San Francisco: Jossey-Bass.

Maurana, C., & Goldenberg, K. (1996). A successful academic-community partnership to improve the public's health. *Academic Medicine, 71*(5), 425–431.

Seifer, S., Connors, K., & O'Neil, E. (1996). Combining service and learning in partnership with communities. *Academic Medicine, 71*, (5), 527.

Resources

BOOKS, ARTICLES, AUTHORS

Bandura, A. (1977). *Social learning theory*. Englewood Cliffs: Prentice-Hall.

Berson, J. S. (1994). A marriage made in heaven: Community colleges and service learning. *Community College Journal, 64*(6), 14–19.

Coles, R. (1993). *The call of service*. Boston: Houghton Mifflin.

Dewey, J. (1916). *Democracy and education*. New York: The Free Press.

Dewey, J. (1938). *Experience and education*. New York: Collier Books.

Ellis, S. J. & Noyes, K. H. (1978). *By the people: A history of Americans as volunteers*. Philadelphia: Energize Books.

Hedin, D., & Conrad, P. (1987). Service: A pathway to knowledge. *Community Education Journal, 15*(1), 10–14.

Jacoby, B. (1996). *Service-learning in higher education: Concepts and practices*. San Francisco: Jossey-Bass Publishers.

Keeton, M. T. & Associates (1977). *Experiential learning: Rationale, characteristics, and assessment*. San Francisco: Jossey-Bass.

Kendall, J. C. (1990). *Combining service and learning: A resource book for community and public service*. Raleigh, NC: National Society for Experiential Education.

Kendall, J. C., Duley, J. S., Permaul, J. S., Rubin, S., & Little, T. (1986). *Strengthening experiential education within your institution*. Raleigh, NC: National Society for Internships and Experiential Education.

Kolb, D. (1984). *Experiential learning*. Englewood Cliffs, NJ: Prentice-Hall.

Lepler, M. (1996). Service learning benefits students, communities. *Nurse Week, 9*(4), 1, 22.

Schon, D. (1983). *The reflective practitioner: How professionals think in action*. New York: Basic.

Schon, D. (1987). *Educating the reflective practitioner*. San Francisco: Jossey-Bass.

Seifer, S. D., Murtha, S., & Connors, K. (1996). Service-learning in health professions education: Barriers, facilitators, and strategies for success. In B. Taylor (Ed.), *Expanding boundaries: Serving and learning* (pp. 36–41). Washington, DC: Corporation for National Service.

Sigmon, R. L. (1979). Service-learning: Three principles. *Synergist National Center for Service Learning Action, 8*(1), 9–11.

Silcox, H. C. (1993). *A how to guide to reflection: Adding cognitive learning to community service programs*. Philadelphia: Brighton Press.

Stanton, T. (1987). Service learning: Groping toward a definition. *Experiential Education, 12*(1), 2, 4.

ORGANIZATIONS

Campus Compact, c/o Brown University, Box 1975
Providence, RI, 02912
e-mail: campus@compact.org

Campus Outreach Opportunity League (COOL)
1531 P Street, NW, Suite LL, Washington, DC 20005

Community-Campus Partnerships for Health
1388 Sutter Street, Suite 805
San Francisco, CA 94109
http://futurehealth.ucsf.edu

Corporation for National Service
1201 New York Avenue, NW
Washington, DC 20525
http://www.nationalservice.org

The Council of Independent Colleges
One Dupont Circle, Suite 320
Washington, DC 20036
e-mail: cic@cic.nche.edu

National Society for Experiential Education
3509 Haworth Drive, Suite 207
Raleigh, NC 27609-7229
http://www.nsee.org

International Partnership for Service-Learning
815 Second Avenue, Suite 315
New York, NY 10017–4594

INTERNET

American Association of Community Colleges
http://www.aacc.nche.edu

National Service-Learning Cooperative Clearinghouse
http://www.nicsl.coled.umn.edu

Nursing Network Forum
http://www.access.digex.net

Service-Learning home page
http://csf.colorado.edu.sl

The Pew Charitable Trusts:Health and Human Services
http://www.pewtrusts.com/docs/hlthhum.html

Consent for Evaluation of Service-Learning Activity

The need for an evaluation of the service- learning activity components of my course has been fully explained to me. I understand data collected will be used for internal and external program reports. I also understand that at some future time results from this evaluation may be published. I have been informed that any information collected will only be reported as group data and at no time will my name be connected to the evaluation data report. My anonymity and confidentiality will be maintained.

Student Signature   Date

Faculty Signature   Date

Qualitative Evaluation

A TIME FOR REFLECTION

AGENCY: _____ COURSE: _____ DATE: _____

1. Describe the following:

    What expectations or myths did you have prior to the experience?

    The most enjoyable aspect of your experience?

    The most frustrating aspect of your experience?

    The most surprising aspect of your experience?

    What did you learn about yourself?

    What did you learn about the health care system/nursing?

    What did you learn about society?

    What did you like/dislike about the community agency?

    What needs did the clients have?

    Did this experience change your ideas of, or approaches to, caring for people?

    Did you feel useful as a volunteer?

2. Describe how this service learning added to your academic life.
    How did it affect your personal life?

Quantitative Service-Learning Evaluation

COURSE NAME & NUMBER _____ SEMESTER & YEAR _____

Please circle the response that best describes your agreement with the statement:

1. The service I did through this class influenced my career plans and goals for the future.
   A   B   C   D
   Strongly Agree   Agree   Disagree   Strongly Disagree

2. I feel the service I did through this class was not at all beneficial to the community.
   A   B   C   D
   Strongly Agree   Agree   Disagree   Strongly Disagree

3. I felt I would have learned more from this class if there were more time spent in the classroom instead of doing service in the community.
   A   B   C   D
   Strongly Agree   Agree   Disagree   Strongly Disagree

4. My course-related learning was enhanced by the service-learning requirements.
   A   B   C   D
   Strongly Agree   Agree   Disagree   Strongly Disagree

5. Service-learning in this course enriched classroom discussion with my peers which I found very helpful.
   A   B   C   D
   Strongly Agree   Agree   Disagree   Strongly Disagree

6. The idea of combining service to the community and university course work should be practiced in more classes at the University of Scranton.
   A   B   C   D
   Strongly Agree   Agree   Disagree   Strongly Disagree

7. This class made me more interested in serving my community than before.
   A   B   C   D
   Strongly Agree   Agree   Disagree   Strongly Disagree

8. Service-learning helped me better understand my role as a resource to the community and the community as a resource to me.

A   B   C   D
Strongly Agree   Agree   Disagree   Strongly Disagree

9. Service-learning helped me examine my values in relation to cultural differences, norms and beliefs of society.

A   B   C   D
Strongly Agree   Agree   Disagree   Strongly Disagree

10. The information presented to me in class and during orientation was sufficient enough for me to begin my service immediately and without much hesitation.

A   B   C   D
Strongly Agree   Agree   Disagree   Strongly Disagree

Program Planning Sample

Course Number	Number of Students Enrolled	Discipline Involved	Goals/Objectives/Content	Setting and Service Learning Components	Timeline
Nursing 140 Introduction to Nursing Concepts	53	Nursing Majors Only	Introduction of core concepts related to nursing as well as the philosophy and conceptual framework of the nursing department. Core concepts explored include client, environment, health, nursing, and health patterns. Historical philosophical and social development of nursing and the role of the professional nurse is addressed. Health and the health continuum are discussed in terms of the broader perspective of human persons, their physiological, psychological, developmental and sociocultural modes. Students are introduced to the concepts of service-learning and given the opportunity to integrate these concepts into their professional learning activities. Students are introduced to the nursing process as it relates to the development of cognitive, interpersonal, and psychomotor skills to assist clients to attain and maintain an optimal level of health.	Each student will chose one of the following activities for their service-learning experience: A. Peer HIV/AIDS Educator Course B. Hospice Volunteer Program C. Geriatric Facility Volunteer. The student will spend a minimum of 15 hours directly involved in one of the above community services. The needs of the project will direct the allocation of these hours.	Year 1 (Academic Year 1995–1996)
Nursing 261 Nursing Related to Health Patterns	55	Nursing Majors Only	Focus on the professional nurses' role in promoting the individual's health status utilizing developmental, physiological, psychological, and sociocultural dimensions of adaptive health patterns. Development of beginning nursing skills and procedures.	The setting and service-learning activities will be developed to address critical issues in the local community that are consistent with our three pronged approaches to focus on Intergenerational needs, Care of the Terminally Ill, and HIV/AIDS Education.	Year 2 (Academic Year 1996–1997)

continued

continued

Course Number	Number of Students Enrolled	Discipline Involved	Goals/Objectives/Content	Setting and Service Learning Components	Timeline
Nursing 380 Nursing the Individual	48	Nursing Majors Only	Focus on the professional nurses' role as caregiver, advocate, and teacher in restoring the physiological and psychosocial adaptive responses of the individual experiencing alterations in the health patterns of self-perception, self-concept, sleep-rest, and activity-exercise. Emphasis placed on the planning and implementation of the nursing process in meeting health needs.	The setting and service-learning activities will be developed to address critical issues in the local community that are consistent with our three pronged approaches to focus on Intergenerational needs, Care of the Terminally Ill, and HIV/AIDS Education	Year 2 (Academic Year 1996–1997)
Nursing 381 Nursing the Individual and Family	48	Nursing Majors Only	Focus on the professional nurse's role as caregiver, advocate and teacher in restoring the physiological and psychosocial adaptive responses of the individual experiencing alterations in the health patterns of self-perception, self-concept, sleep-rest, and activity-exercise. Emphasis placed on the planning and implementation of the nursing process in meeting health needs.	The setting and service-learning activities will be developed to address critical issues in the local community that are consistent with our three-pronged approaches to focus on Intergenerational needs, Care of the Terminally Ill, and HIV/AIDS Education	Year 3 (Academic Year 1997–1998)

					Year 1 (Academic Year 1995–1996)
Nursing 480 Nursing the Individual, Family, Community	36	Nursing Majors Only	Focus on the professional nurse's role as caregiver, advocate and teacher in promoting and restoring adaptive responses of the individual, family and community experiencing alternations in the health patterns of elimination, cognitive-perceptual, coping-stress tolerance, and value belief. Emphasis is placed on the planning and implementation phases of the nursing process in meeting health needs. Students are provided with the opportunity to expand their understanding of the concept of "service-learning" within their professional activities.	The setting and service-learning activities will be developed to address critical issues in the local community that are consistent with our three-pronged approaches to focus on Intergenerational needs, Care of the Terminally Ill, and HIV/AIDS Education	
Nursing 482 Synthesis of Nursing Concepts	36	Nursing Majors Only	Focus on the professional nurse's role as leader-manager in promoting, restoring and maintaining adaptive responses in individuals experiencing complex alterations in health patterns. Continued use of the nursing process to implement and evaluate nursing care of the individual, family, community and groups in collaboration with the nursing and interdisciplinary health teams.	The setting and service-learning activities will be developed to address critical issues in the local community that are consistent with our three pronged approaches to focus on Intergenerational needs, Care of the Terminally Ill, and HIV/AIDS Education	First year following end of grant (Academic Year 1998–1999)

continued

continued

Course Number	Number of Students Enrolled	Discipline Involved	Goals/Objectives/Content	Setting and Service Learning Components	Timeline
Nursing 100 Family Health	250 (per year/ multiple sections)	Non-nursing Majors	Concepts and principals related to the promotion and maintenance of optimal family health. Considers factors pertinent to health needs and health practices throughout the life cycle.	The setting and service-learning activities will be developed to address critical issues in the local community that are consistent with our three-pronged approaches to focus on Intergenerational needs, Care of the Terminally Ill, and HIV/AIDS Education	Year 2 (Academic Year 1996–1997)
Incorporate Service Learning into Graduate Program	approximately 25 students per academic year (full and part time students)	Graduate Nursing Majors Only	Prepare advanced practice nurses who assess, diagnose, and treat complex individual and family health problems to improve health outcomes. The nurse practitioner is prepared to provide primary health care to families with a focus in rural settings.	The setting and service-learning activities will be developed to address critical issues in the local community that are consistent with our three-pronged approaches to focus on Intergenerational needs, Care of the Terminally Ill, and HIV/AIDS Education	First year following end of grant (Academic Year 1998–1999)

Begin Development of at least one interdisciplinary course that involves service-learning	Approximately 30 students per year	Students from all majors	Focus on interdisciplinary health care in the community	The setting and service-learning activities will be developed to address critical issues in the local community that are consistent with our three-pronged approaches to focus on Intergenerational needs, Care of the Terminally Ill, and HIV/AIDS Education	First Year beyond the end of the grant period. (Academic Year 1998–1999)

Sample Program Design: Integration of Service-Learning into Introductory Nursing Course

INTRODUCTION TO NURSING CONCEPTS

This is the first required nursing course taken by freshmen nursing majors. Generally, there are no more 55 students in the class. Current content for this particular course is related to issues pertinent to nursing, nursing history, problem solving, and the conceptual framework that supports the entire curriculum for the Department of Nursing at the University of Scranton. The setting and service-learning component for the course was developed over several years. The major course project in this class was as follows:

Each student will choose one of the following activities (A or B) for the major course project (25% of the final course grade).

A. A Service-learning activity:

Students will engage in *one* of the following:
    a. Peer HIV/AIDS Educator course
    b. Hospice Volunteer Program
    c. Long-Term Care facility volunteer
    d. Hospital Volunteer Program

The student will spend a minimum of 15 hours directly involved in one of the above community services. The needs of the project will direct the allocation of these hours. For example, the HIV/AIDS peer education course may be done in blocks of 4-5 hours each. Each student will design the allocation of the hours in consultation with the Service-Learning Coordinator and community agency personnel. Critical reflection will be a part of each service-learning project.

Requirements:

1. Attend the Orientation Period for the service-learning activity (varies with each agency).
2. Fulfill the assigned hours (30 pts.)
3. Prepare and submit an annotated bibliography of 5 articles (20 pts.)
4. Maintain a "dialogue journal" to be shared with the community agency contact person and the course instructor after each service contact (25 pts.)
5. Prepare a written report to be shared with the community agency and the class (25 pts.)

OR

B. Issue Paper:

Choose an issue in nursing applicable to practice, education, or future role development. Identify your own position and reflect on this in a scholarly writing style. The suggested length of the paper is 10–15 pages and is to follow the APA format. The outline for the paper is:

1. Introduction and abstract (10 points)
2. Analysis of the issue: (50 points)
    A. Describe the issue
    B. What factors influence the issue

       C. Propose resolutions
       D. Propose implementation strategies
       E. Identify future implications
       F. Evaluate the impact on nursing
    3. Summary (10 points)
    4. Format and style of writing (30 points)

Sample Program Design: Integration of Service-Learning into Senior Level Nursing Course

NURSING THE INDIVIDUAL/FAMILY/COMMUNITY

This course enrolls on the average 40 students per academic year, although there is the possibility of having as many as 55 students. The current content for this course is related to Community Health Nursing and complex medical-surgical problems. The service-learning component for the course is completed in the following project:

Community Assessment Project/Service-Learning Activity
(10% of course grade)

Students will analyze a health care need within the community through service-learning. The project will consist of four sections: a community profile, a plan for intervention, a description of the intervention, and an evaluation of the implementation by:

A. Demonstrating certification by the American Red Cross in Disaster Nursing, or
B. Preparing an oral presentation to be given to the community agency and the class based upon a search of the literature and a personal journal kept during the project on the topic of homelessness, or
C. Identifying a problem within the community (for example, childhood safety, drug and alcohol abuse, environmental hazards, access to health care). Students choosing this option will:
   1. Identify the problem;
   2. Interview community leaders;
   3. Determine available resources in the community;
   4. Identify strengths and weaknesses in the community;
   5. Plan a community response to the identified problem;
   6. Implement the plan; and
   7. Report the results, including implications and recommendations.

Each student will spend a minimum of 15 hours directly involved in a specific community service. Allocation of the hours will be designed in consultation with the service-learning coordinator and community agency personnel. Critical reflection will be a part of each service-learning project.

Index

(Page numbers followed by "t" indicate tables.)